My Adventures in

Rural Surgery of India

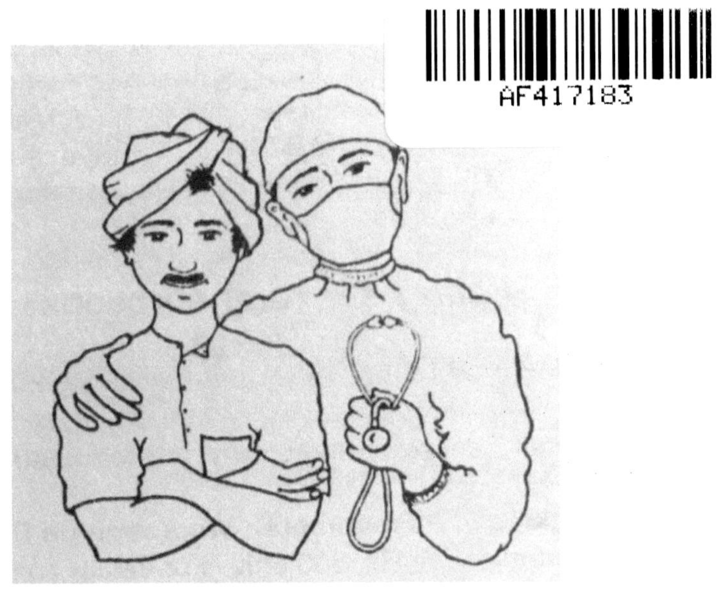

Memoirs of Dr R. D. Prabhu

ISBN-13 : 979-8889511632

2nd Edition 2025

Made with 🤍 on the Notion Press Platform

www.notionpress.com

ॐ सर्वे भवन्तु सुखिनः

सर्वे सन्तु निरामयाः ।

सर्वे भद्राणि पश्यन्तु

मा कश्चिद्दुःखभाग्भवेत् ।।

ॐ शान्तिः शान्तिः शान्तिः

May all be happy

May all be free of illnesses

My all see happy bodings

May no one become unhappy

Peace for all

This book is dedicated to all those invisible practitioners in small towns and rural places who, taking all risks, strive to deliver appropriate, affordable broad based surgical care to their communities.

Contents

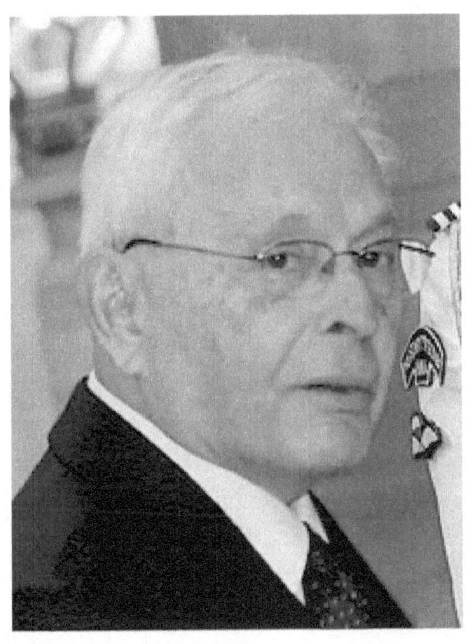

Foreword

I consider it an honour and a privilege to be requested to write a foreword for this book by Dr. R.D.Prabhu ('My Adventures in Rural Surgery of India'). Spread over six decades, I have been a Consultant Surgeon at a Tertiary Care Hospital and a Professor at Teaching Hospital in Mumbai. Fortuitously, I was gifted the God given opportunity to travel for decades (from 1975) to small town and rural India in pursuit of my mission to spread diagnostic laparoscopy and later operative laparoscopy. I have travelled ostensibly to teach and spread laparoscopy but every visit I made over rural India, I returned humbled, educated, inspired by the quality, courage, sacrifice of the Indian Rural Surgeon.

During my early years of travel through rural India I met some of the pioneers of Rural Surgeons in India who struggled and broke new ground to give quality, standards, dignity and authenticity to rural surgery in India. One of the Founding Fathers of rural surgery was Dr. R.D.Prabhu.

This book is written in the simple, homely, unpretentious style of a down to earth rural surgeon, who tells of his youth, his doctor father and more importantly, it tells of his thorough grounding in General Surgery over several years, most of it in the UK. Apart from training in General Surgery, in anticipation of his desire to serve the poor in India, he got experience in specialties required for practice in rural areas – casualty and emergency, urology, plastic surgery, ENT, orthopaedic surgery and so on. In an era where Professors in Teaching Hospitals inculcate the importance and the need of sub and super specialization to their students, Dr. Prabhu and his colleagues feel that for the majority of Indians and their surgical problems, the ultimate super-specialty is wide-based general surgery. They could trephine for an intra-cranial bleed, drain an empyema, resect an intestinal gangrene, perform a Caesarean section and treat compound fractures. They were dedicated to doing this despite meagre finances, restricted equipment, not a single qualified support staff, impossible working conditions because they knew they were the last bastion of poor who had travelled long distances to reach them. Their financial returns may be meagre, but their inner joys and satisfaction are bountiful. This is the quiet, almost hidden story woven through the pages of this book, the qualities of innovation, improvisation, but most of all the quality of love, empathy, care and devotion to their patients, qualities one sees being eroded elsewhere.

Dr. Prabhu and his equally endowed colleagues created the Association of Rural surgeons of India (ARSI), which has given identity, cohesion, fellowship, education to rural surgeons. There are thousands of rural surgeons. I find it very disappointing that every rural surgeon is not a member of this Association. In numbers and unity is strength. The organized, united rural surgical community would be a vibrant force to reckon with, to stand up to ignorant, clueless orders passed by courts or regulatory bodies, ignorant of their working conditions or commitment for the welfare of their patients.

This book tells the story of the surgeons who are the back bone of Indian Surgery.

Dr. Tehemton E. Udwadia,   31/10/2022

MS, FCPS, FRCS(Eng), FRCS(Edin), FICS(Hon), FACS,FAMS
Padma Bhushan (2017)
Padma Shri (2006)
Father Of Laparoscopic Surgery in India
B. C. Roy Award

Preface

It never occurred to me to write a book. My close friends at the Association of Rural Surgeons of India (ARSI) have written some books, but I never imagined that I would too. Some well-wishers like Dr Nabhojit Roy and later Dr Nakul Raykar from Lancet Global Health asked me to pass on my experience to the next generation, and later Eric Kim and Rohini Dutta's write-up in *BMJ Global Health* (See page 161) urged me on. After some more encouragement and coaxing by Dr Kavery Nambisan, I became serious about it. If my experiences would be of help to at least a few others, it would be worth the effort.

> Lives of great men all remind us
> We can make our lives sublime,
> And, departing, leave behind us
> Footprints on the sands of time;
>
> Footprints, that perhaps another,
> Sailing o'er life's solemn main,
> A forlorn and shipwrecked brother,
> Seeing, shall take heart again.
>
> -   Psalm of Life- H. W. Longfellow

I thought, leaving a few of my "footprints on the sands of time" too may help someone or the other in future, like how I myself learnt by reading the experiences of other surgeons. Experiences of others are valuable teachers when it comes to rural surgery – because no textbook prepares you for it!

Our elders rightly said:

आचार्यात् पादमादत्ते पादं शिष्यः स्वमेधया ।
सब्रह्मचारिभ्यः पादं पादं कालक्रमेण च ॥

"A quarter of what we learn is from teachers, schools and colleges, a quarter from one's own studying, a quarter from colleagues, and the remaining quarter from experience gained with time"

In this book, I write about my learning from teachers and consultants I worked with, from my colleagues and from my own experiences, performing surgeries in a small Indian town with very limited facilities. I prefer to call it 'Rural Surgery of India', but it is quite similar to the 'Global Surgery' that Lancet Global Health is trying to implement across the globe by 2030. According to *BMJ Global Health*, Global Surgery is the term adopted to describe a rapidly developing multidisciplinary field aiming to provide improved and equitable surgical care across international health systems. The Lancet Commission on Global Surgery, which brings together many high-profile institutions from across the world, wishes to make governments realise that surgery is an indispensable, indivisible part of basic health care provision, and to make the required surgical and anaesthesia facilities available to all, including the low- and middle-income groups. In many ways, this is similar to what we practiced in Shimoga for nearly half a century – a kind of interdisciplinary, inexpensive way of treatment that is within the reach of all. The adventure that we called Rural Surgery of India is the Global Surgery of the future that Lancet Global Health visualises. In essence, in rural surgery, giving relief and/or saving a life is more important than any academic aspect of surgery.

This book is about the many occasions when academics took a back seat. It is about the difficulties I faced as a surgeon in a small town, as also the rigors of training that I had to go through to face them. It is difficult to imagine the level to which small towns and villages in India lack basic facilities and manpower for surgical care. There are no easy answers in colleges or books to solve these difficulties we face. The Association of Rural Surgeons of India (ARSI) found that almost all rural surgeons face similar difficulties, and interestingly, they all find their own unique ways of overcoming them. Besides, they may even have to use an old method or even bend the laws a little! Their ultimate aim is to give relief to the patient, reach the unreached.

I have met in recent past, some specialists and professors whose opinions reveal their lack of empathy and ignorance of the state of health(surgical) care in rural India. One Orthopaedic Professor (Davangere) had said "Why do you want to teach orthopaedics to rural surgeons? Send all orthopaedic patients to us (Med. College) and we will manage them....". He ignored the "Golden hour" that will be lost by the time patient reaches Med. College. One Prof of Anaesthesia (Kerala) said "Only Prof. of Anaesthesia should give anaesthesia in rural hospitals....." Do we have so many anaesthetists to go rural hospitals? One obstetrician in Udupi Govt. Hospital performed thousands of Caesarean sections under local anaesthesia because she did not have anaesthetists to help her in her earlier days! One Prof. of Surgery in Mangalore said that he "always had an anaesthetist stand by in his O.T. whenever he performed surgery under Local Anaesthesia..." What about thousands and more dentists working with local anaesthesia day in and day out? I have had to ignore such professorial 'opinions' for the ease of function and to help the patient in time. A rural surgeon can attend to farm accidents, road accidents etc. in time saving a limb, lives, babies perhaps, saving blood loss, and mortality and morbidity that are likely during the time lost in transportation to medical colleges.

Many who know about this, like Dr. Balu Sankaran, Dr. N.H.Antia, Dr. T.E. Udwadia, Dr Ramesh Pai of Hyderabad, neuro-surgeon Dr. Ramamurthy (Chennai) and many others felt the rural surgeons form the main force for the present and future Bharat's health care!   Opinions of judiciary, given after months of deliberations too show how they too fail to realise how difficult it is to decide "on the spot" and "immediately" in many tricky situations threatening life. It is said that a judiciary involved in sanctioning blood bank rules was there in the hospital where his own daughter was admitted for delivery. When she needed blood transfusion urgently, he was taken a back at the race for time to procure that lifesaving unit of blood! He is said to have confessed that blood bank rules might have been passed in a hurry! So it appears to me that these adversities make it far more difficult to practice surgery in a small town than to practice in a big hospital in a city. It is hard enough to perform surgery in a well-equipped hospital, but performing the same in a rural setup is nothing short of an adventure!

During the life time of every surgeon, rural or urban, he comes across surgical problems that were never taught or faced during his college of training career. Yet he is required to deal with them to the best of his ability, as it is often seen that the surgeon nearby is the last hope for the patient. Urban surgeons may have colleagues nearby to help him out but not so for rural surgeon! This may happen once only in his lifetime but that one time may save a life! I had some patients where I had to refer to the books or innovate; some of them were unique and memorable. It is mainly because of such bold initiatives shown by rural surgeons that rural and small town surgeons continue to be relevant. Unfortunately, and it is a pity that, people and even the ignorant judiciary ignore all the good work done and the lives saved by the doctor over the years only to victimize him for some unintended error. I too have faced such situations, where I had to search for solutions in books or innovate; some of them being unique and memorable. Besides, conventionally, General Surgery means treating all surgical problems from the abdomen, perineum, lumps and bumps etc. but it was not long before I realized that I had to manage problems from other branches of surgery; for example, drain an empyema, incise a quinsy, set fractures, reduce dislocation of a joint, remove large stones in urinary bladder and so on. Wide based training in the UK was very helpful to deal with all of this. Such bold and satisfying challenges motivate rural and small-town surgeons to continue working despite all odds.

I have not provided the accurate dates, ages, and other surgical details of each case. But being so exceptionally interesting, they are still etched in my memory. I have penned down the important aspects of such cases. Perhaps what is in words should be there in pictures too, but I could not take pictures of all my work earlier as I never dreamt then of publishing them at some point in my life.

It is difficult to write research papers based on a rural surgeon's data, which has many shortcomings. Everyone would want to know numbers, statistics, double blind studies, investigations, references, and so on. I never had these – yet I managed to produce a couple of papers. One of them was on surgery without antibiotics in a rural hospital. I have included it in this book.

I hope this book – the experiences, the cases and the solutions adopted then – will give other doctors who practice in rural India a chance to reminisce about their own experiences; and the younger generation an idea of what it is like to practice in rural India. Medical practice in rural India throws surprise after surprise every single day, yet rewards you with the utmost satisfaction.

It is my belief that Rural Surgery of India (though it was not known by that name earlier) started with Sushruta, or even before him. I do not know much about who taught, who learnt and who practiced it. But if a potter (*kumbhar*) could repair a cut nose (referred to in the chapter on surgery without antibiotics), Indian Rural Surgery was indeed being practiced at all levels. It perhaps evolved according to the needs of the patients in those days, nurtured by the efforts of the *vaidyas*. Then came the outsiders, who tried hard to establish their own superiority over Ayurveda. This new Western medicine, no doubt, was far superior and gave good results, quickly. But it was not easily available to commoners, leave alone the poor.

As far as my memory goes back, when a trained surgeon was not available, a doctor with a basic MBBS degree could give relief or save lives by unconventional methods (incision of an abscess), resorting to unorthodox techniques (Colle's fracture reduction), ignoring modern surgical protocols (child delivery without gloves), or even breaking blood bank rules (auto-transfusion)! Professors and colleges neither condoned nor encouraged such practices. Yet, conscientious practitioners persevered with such life-saving adventures.

When we decided to form the Association of Rural Surgeons of India, we could not decide what defines 'rural' in rural surgery. So, we concluded that it denotes the conditions found in villages or small towns. We further developed it into 'Rural Surgery of India', because each country has its own culture, people, conditions and methods that influence the surgeon, and we are influenced by patients of India that is Bharat.

So, in reverence to Sushruta, father of surgery in India, and perhaps in the world too, to retain our national pride and identity, we should perhaps continue calling it Rural Surgery of India, until a better name is found. And that is exactly what it was, during my practice from 1970 to 2015!

Dr R. D. Prabhu

Acknowledgments

I began writing this book on the suggestion of the Lancet Global Health Group (LGH). I penned down some of my experiences, and they liked it. Then, things just stalled. I would have given it up there, but suddenly, Eric Kim and Rohini Dutta of LGH published a write-up about me in BMJ Global Health. That revived my interest in the book. Again, there was a long lull and I wondered if my book would see the light of day, ever!

Suddenly, two personalities appeared on the scene. I had asked Dr Kavery Nambisan, author of A Luxury Called Health, for an honest opinion of whether this book deserved publishing, and she replied with an emphatic yes. Even more encouraging was Dr Tehempton Udwadia, considered the father of Indian Laparoscopic Surgery and also author of More Than Just Surgery. He felt that my book is a must-read for all doctors, and encouraged me to publish it soon!

I am grateful to all these people for encouraging me to go ahead with my book. My only regret is that I could not publish it fast enough to hand over one copy to him when he was alive!

I am immensely thankful to Janani Gopalakrishnan Vikram for editing my amateurish writing into a readable book. My wife Usha's presence can be felt in all the pages of this book. Neither our practice in Shimoga nor this book can even be imagined without her!

Then, there are all my family members – young and old – who have played their role to perfection! Vivek, our son, has contributed immensely in many different ways. Our daughter

Suneela, son-in-law Harish, daughter-in-law Vandana and the grandchildren have together made this book a family project, helping me with their timely comments and suggestions for improvement.

I happily appreciate their support and contributions!

Introduction

Reflecting on my career as a surgeon, I am very happy with some of my achievements and also sorry about the inevitable failures. While a lot has been achieved, some things could have been better. I know I cannot go back and make amends, but I cannot help but think, "If only I could…". However, I honestly feel that I have been immensely satisfied being instrumental in giving relief, reducing suffering and morbidities, and saving lives of so many.

Rural Surgery is like our corner grocery store. It is there for anything we want in an emergency. Though not as dazzling as a supermarkt or departmental store and the shop looks small and in a 'mess' unlike a well arranged and well stocked departmental store, one gets everything there; from grocery, toiletry, cosmetics, stationary, sweets, vegetables, fruits, bakery products and what not. You may not see the item on the shelf but he finds it behind some or other bottle, in the corner of shelf etc. Some stores in villages even sell petrol in bottles for those two-wheel owners. Likewise, a rural hospital and surgeon though not comparable to any corporate or teaching hospital, is there to help one in an emergency to save a life, tide over an emergency, buy time till you reach a higher center and so on. In fact, if the rural surgeon is conversant with the 44 essential skills selected by W.H.O. and the Disease Control Priorities (United Nations 2015) listed earlier, he may be able to manage most of the emergencies by himself! This admirable entrepreneurship of a rural surgeon is in adapting a technology of developed countries whose per capita income is ten times or more than that of India!

I grew up in a small town, little bigger than a village! Ankola, in North Kanara, Karnataka (earlier to 1956 it was in the Bombay presidency). It is a small town, a little bigger than a village! So when I grow up, I wanted to be a helpful 'dacter' in a similar town too, to be of help to people living in such places. In this book, I recollect the severe odds and constraints that my wife Usha and I faced while setting up our surgical practice in a similar small town, and the great satisfaction we got despite all the difficulties faced. Our surgical techniques might have been the same as those practiced by others elsewhere at that time, but we often had to improvise minor changes and innovations to overcome the absence of facilities. That meant compromising latest practices, but in the interest of the patients, it was better than doing nothing. Such practices were accepted in our times, by patients who implicitly trusted their doctors. Now, with Google at everyone's fingertips and tempting Consumer Protection Act (CPA) compensations, this trust is disappearing; and surgeons too are hesitant to take risks even with good intentions! I believe that the patient stands to lose here.

I witnessed how bold compromises had to be made when my uncle had his wrist fracture set right. Such compromises help rural surgeons overcome the lack of facilities, and the end justifies the means. An elderly uncle of mine sustained a Colle's fracture of his left hand. I was a student then, hoping to go to a medical college. We had to go to the district surgeon in the District Hospital in Karwar, some distance away for X-Ray and treatment. I was permitted to accompany him as I wanted to be a doctor in the future. An X-ray of his wrist confirmed the clinical diagnosis. Now, the problem was that there was no anaesthetist in the hospital on that day! Postponing the treatment was not practical either. So, the surgeon said the only feasible alternative was to try and reduce the fracture with local anaesthesia, a very poor substitute for general anaesthesia! My uncle's accompanying doctor (my father) agreed to this and explained to the uncle that there is bound to be some discomfort with such anaesthesia, and he would have to bear some pain too; however, it was imperative to reduce the fracture and apply a plaster cast on the same day.

The surgeon organised the procedure. In those days, the plaster of paris (POP) bandage rolls had to be prepared fresh in hospitals, by sprinkling plaster of paris powder on cut lengths of gauze bandage, and then rolling layers of the bandage with plaster powder between them. In fact, in my early years in Shimoga, we too prepared POP bandages in this manner. When everything was ready, the patient was made to lie on a table. The surgeon wanted two people to apply traction to the forearm, one holding the elbow and arm, and the other holding the hand. I was made to hold the elbow. The district surgeon then took a generous quantity (I do not remember the strength, volume or name) of the local anaesthetic, and injected it directly into the haematoma of the fracture site! My uncle, who was moaning and groaning when we had his forearm in our grips, soon stopped moaning and was happy to be free of pain. The surgeon then took hold of the wrist and manipulated the fracture blindly – it was pre C-arm days. My uncle suddenly groaned loudly – so loudly that I swooned, and actually had a blackout with cold sweat on my forehead and face. I was still holding the arm, unaware of the completion of the procedure. Someone noticed my state and quickly relieved me. By this time, the plaster cast was applied and my uncle was quiet. The forearm was fixed in a sling and we returned home.

This was my first experience of the use of local anaesthetic at a fracture site. Nobody uses it now for fear of infection; I have only read about it in literature. This was an example of a nineteenth-century procedure being used in the twentieth century! Such situations are bound to crop up even today in a rural surgeon's life. When giving relief to the patient becomes a priority, compromised treatment comes to the rescue, even though it may appear crude, non-academic and unorthodox, and be looked down upon by peers and academic-minded colleagues! In the early days of my practice in Shimoga, when we did not have an anaesthetist, I too have had to resort to this method to reduce a Colle's fracture. Thankfully, there was no complication. Of course, the anaesthesia is not as complete as a general anaesthesia; the patient does feel some pain. But fracture dis-impaction and reduction can be achieved.

Coping with Inadequate Facilities

When we decided to start giving oral polio drops to children in 1971-72, they were available only from a chemist in Bangalore, 300km away. Cold chain equipment was not available and that Bangalore chemist did not have a cold chain to deliver the drops in Shimoga. As was the practice with other medical practitioners, I had to go to Bangalore with a thermos flask filled with ice cubes and bring the vials of polio-drops in it – a journey that took around six hours each way. Unused drops had to be stored in an ordinary kitchen refrigerator! I was aware of the defects of such cold storage, but there was no better alternative. We used these drops for our own children too, just as for others who came to us; the only alternative was leaving these children exposed to polio virus! Inefficiency of our method came to light when our son developed weakness in his right leg – probably an early non-paralytic stage of polio-myelitis. However, we were very relieved when he recovered completely, with only splinting and total rest.

Similarly, when a person came with a fracture of the thigh bone, I had to treat him with traction and bed rest (a method of earlier days) instead of the latest internal fixation of the bone, because my nursing home – just like any other in Shimoga – was not equipped for that surgery.

Dr. Sitanath De FRCS, a friend of mine in Jhargram, West Bengal, performed an old procedure of joining the common bile duct to the gut (Chole-docho-duodenostomy, an old method) for common bile duct obstruction with calculi (stones); because his patient could not afford to go to Kolkata for advanced procedures like exploration of the common bile duct. "That is an old method, old method" shouted one professor! Though my friend was more than qualified to perform the newer 'exploration', he did not have the facilities, anesthetist and equipment for it, and had to resort to a method of the earlier century for the sake of his patient.

In this book, I have not written much about the latest surgical procedures that I have performed, but mostly about how I had to resort to older techniques under the circumstances.

Newer technology is, no doubt, vastly superior, but it needs costly equipment and facilities. X-ray was useful for us. Computed Tomography (CT) scan is superior, and is available in most places now. Magnetic Resonance Imaging (MRI) gives even more, and better information. However, the cost of extra information with each method keeps mounting. So, the treating doctor has to consider the relevance of the extra information against the patient's finances. The patient's circumstances will also decide the need for being treated locally, without upsetting his family life and profession, vis-à-vis being treated in a faraway place where newer technology is available. If an X-ray gives all the information that is needed, it does not make economic sense to ask for a CT scan or MRI

Jungle Surgery

My medical education was in Bombay (now Mumbai), India, and surgical training was in the United Kingdom. The visit to UK made me aware of the disparities between surgery as shown in textbooks, surgery that we actually practiced in our medical college hospitals, and the surgery that was practiced in British National Health Scheme (NHS) hospitals at that time. Even though the actual surgical procedures were similar, many things were different. In India, as Sadguru Jaggi Vasudev said in a recent media interview, "Some people live in the twenty-first century, while the rest of the country lives in the twentieth or even nineteenth centuries!" Besides, the treatment in UK hospitals is free to the patient, tailored to the needs of their people. In India, that is Bharat, we try to copy western practice of health care ignoring the cost factor. We differ in many aspects of our lives, from food habits to behaviour. But what we rural surgeons practice is more like the *"jungle surgery"* described later in this book. We resort to some old method, or modify text-book surgery to make it affordable and to bypass the constraints, are quite at home with chaos, lack of punctuality, lack of respect for social protocols, poor public hygiene, varied food habits, the notorious *'chalta hai'* attitude, and such. The worst is the poverty that interferes with every attempt to give quality treatment. After all, health care costs have to be borne by the patients themselves. If any investigation or medication is beyond the patient's pocket, he or she will just go home without the investigation, and without treatment too!

The contrast between Indian wards and UK wards was palpably obvious. Our ward 'routines', our nursing methods and practices, our protocols, are all so different from those in the UK. So, though the technical side of surgical procedures were similar, the practice of surgery as a whole in UK hospitals was far different from that in our hospitals. In short, I had to re-orient myself to the new system!

Was it better in the UK? Well, yes. Surgery was practiced mostly as written in the books, and if any surgeons deviated from the routine and the results were good, it was accepted by others. In those days, it did not require affirmation from above. Mr. Sanford FRCS, MRCP in Ryhope General Hospital, did not believe in painting tincture iodine on the skin before incising for surgery; he called applying tincture iodine etc. "black magic". Mr. Sanford was right; there was no increase in the incidence of post op. infection rate in his patients, compared to the other surgeon, Mr. Kempsey FRCS who used tincture iodine religiously as was the practice everywhere. When I told about this during FRCS examination, the examiner gracefully accepted Mr. Sanford's practice! How do I know? I had passed that examination. In the U.K. those days, such practices did not require authentication from above. Our Indian teachers, on the other hand, hesitate to step away from the 'trodden path' even when they know an alternative is more beneficial to our patients, like use of sugar for wound dressing (described later in this book).

On my return from the UK to Shimoga in 1970, I could practice the newly-learnt surgical procedures, but it was impossible to bring in other good aspects of the hospital and nursing practices from there. I had not realised at the time that the U.K. economy (1970) was 20 to 25 times more (Rs. 17,600 per capita) than that of India (Rs. 590 per capita). And so, I had to unlearn a lot of what I had learnt and re-adjust to our poverty, lack of facilities and equipment and chaos. That included accepting the inconvenient habits of Indian patients like not keeping appoint-ments, forgetting to bring earlier personal medical notes, ignoring medical instructions and untidiness. An Indian surgeon has to accept such tardiness of Indian patients. Here a surgeon is more connected with his patient, almost 24x7 unlike in the UK where patients do not get to ring up their surgeon. In fact, accepting all that is a step towards success in practice in India. These non-technical aspects of this practice are not usually found in any textbook, but learnt from Indian surgical wards, colleagues and are accepted as normal.

Just to describe the state of medical infrastructure in Shimoga in 1970 to practice surgery, I found myself in a different, older period of time and age altogether. This place did not have a basic clinical laboratory. A retired lab assistant used to read haemoglobin levels using the 'blotting paper' method. We bought Sahli's haemoglobinometer. There was no other lab investigation available. When my brother brought me a German microscope we started doing ourselves differential count of W.B.C.s stool exam and urine microscopy. In the beginning we used hand operated centrifuge. "Blood Bank" did not exist. A staff nurse in the Govt. Hospital would cross match a donor with the patient and collect blood of suitable donor in a bottle for transfusion. Ultrasound, C-arm and CT scans were unheard of. I did not have a cautery unit either, and had to tie individual bleeding points separately. There were no trained nurses; we had to train young girls right from the ground up, including basics like how to give intramuscular injections, how to make beds, feel pulse, how to give enema, what to use in enema fluids, how to roll a bandage, and more. There being fewer nurses in a ward than necessary, it was and is very common in India to see relatives perform many of the 'nursing' duties for the patient. I had to get used to it too.

How does one sterilise the instruments and the linen? An operation theatre (OT) technician of a colleague of mine told us that instruments are sterile after three whistles by the autoclave. I did not believe it. I tried to find the correct way of sterilisation, from the pathology departments of three medical colleges, including my own. Shockingly, all three differed! Fortunately, I had a book on OT procedures. Many may know the process of autoclaving, but most do not know that it is different for steel instruments and for cotton towels! Steel instruments need 30 minutes under 120lbs pressure, i.e., from the time steam escapes from the valve, while cotton towels and linen need 45-60 minutes under 120lbs. For effective sterilisation there is a certain method of packing linen in a drum too; the folded sheets and towels must be placed vertically and not too tightly, so that steam circulates around them freely. I learnt all this from that book. These might not be listed amongst the duties of a surgeon; but a rural surgeon needs to know them.

We had purchased a steam steriliser from a reputed manufacturer in Bombay. I believe they only manufacture but do not test its efficacy! When I tested it with 3M Bowie-Dick autoclave tape, I found that the sterilisation was incomplete. I also found that steam holes on the instrument - drums of the steriliser, were too small. The supplier's technician, who had come to install the steriliser, was speechless; no one had shown him this. I enlarged the holes with a hand drill and now the sterilisation was complete in the stipulated time! I could boldly perform clean surgeries without use of antibiotics!

We could not find any trained OT technicians; I had to train one, Govinda for it. He soon mastered sterilisation procedures, learnt about the instrument and to assist too.

There were no ambulances. Patients came in all types of transport; mostly in horse-drawn 'tongas' (horse carts). The ambulance with the Government Hospital (GH) was used only for transporting patients to a big hospital far away. Worst of all, the "ambulance" was not worth its name. It did not have facilities for patients; it was being used mostly as a delivery van for moving materials.

Most shocking was the fact that we did not have a qualified anaesthetist either, the very basic need for any surgery these days. The Govt. Hospital with most of the speciality departments managed with an assistant surgeon trained in anaesthesia. In the early days I had to send away patients needing surgery under general anaesthesia. Since I could give spinal (regional) anaesthesia, learnt from Dr. Metgud in Davangere, we could perform lower abdominal surgery alone. Later we had to utilise the services of the Govt. Asst. surgeon anaesthetist.

Though the famous Jog Falls was just 100 kilometres away and all the power it generated came to Shimoga before being distributed to the rest of the State, power supply in Shimoga was absolutely unpredictable; there were occasions when we had to use hand-held torches to complete the surgery. Once when lower section Caesarean section was being performed, there was sudden power cut when the baby was about to be extracted. Relatives ran and brought a 'petromax' lamp, one that has a glowing filament. Manual foot suction pump was required to suck out the blood and liquor!

As for the actual surgery, the specialisations were yet to come here, and the old broad-based general surgery was still better-suited to these people.

When I took up my last job in the UK, the consultant knew that I would certainly return to India. He told me that what was practiced in the UK at that time might not be suitable for my practice in India; I needed to learn the appropriate surgery for India, what he called 'jungle surgery'. That was not to insult India, but to make me aware of the reality. After nearly 50 years of that type of surgical practice in India I believe that my practice was more of jungle surgery, now euphemistically called rural surgery (or Global Surgery).

We all know that surgery is far more advanced in the UK; I could learn and earn there. That was one of the reasons why I chose to go to the UK. Working for the NHS and studying in the UK was a good choice. I hoped to bring newer technologies back with me and pass on the benefits to Indian patients. But… jungle surgery was still needed!

The petty politics that ravages India in all its spheres of activities, almost drove me back to the UK. But family bonding held me back. Now, if one were to ask me if my decision to stay back in India was right, I would say emphatically that it was. I could fulfil my dream of being useful to our own people, being near my family, and being of use professionally to many of my relatives. I had a better social standing here compared to what I would have had in the UK, having found a place in our community, a membership in a service organisation like the Rotary Club, and an office in our own ARSI. I could serve our parents, and also bring up our children amidst our own proud cultural traditions. Much more satisfaction was derived after our retirement from practice, when so many satisfied patients expressed their gratitude and respect. Another important thing was that I was able to follow both my passions – general surgery and painting (mainly after retirement). So yes, I did what I had originally dreamed of, and I am happy about it all!

1. Drainage of an Abscess

This was the first surgery I witnessed, and was perhaps key to my choosing this career!

It was during the British Raj, that is, before India got her independence. Healthcare in my district, and perhaps others too, was in shambles. Despite having a Government Hospital, people depended more on efficient private clinics. Surgical care was available only in the district headquarters, far away. You had to go even farther, to Hubli, or preferably to Bombay, for better facilities.

I was young then, maybe eight or 10 years old. Our neighbour had a three- or four-years old boy who was ill; he had an abscess over his knee. Now I know it was probably a pre-patellar bursa abscess. My father, a Licentiate of the College of Physicians and Surgeons (LCPS), was the family's neighbour-cum-doctor. It was obvious to him that the boy needed a surgeon's help. But the whole district had only one surgeon, that too in the district headquarters miles away from our place. Bullock carts were a common mode of travel. For 'long distances' the occasional bus might have been there. Most importantly, the boy's family could not afford the trip to, or the treatment at the district hospital, or even in the local Government Hospital for that matter. So, my father – the boy's doctor – had to do whatever needed to be done.

It was before the days of antibiotics; I am not even sure if any sulphonamides were in use. The abscess became tense and the boy became very ill. The obvious treatment was to let out the pus. One day, my father boiled one of his old-fashioned knives, called a bistoury. In those days, the blades of the scalpel used to be one with the handle. A bistoury blade is curved on its sharp edge, with a very sharp pointed tip. There was no anaesthesia at all, not even an ethyl chloride spray (which we used in the fifties to anaesthetise the patient or the surface of an abscess), or some Ether. The only available accessories were a spirit bottle, tincture of benzoin, iodoform, wet cotton swabs, dry cotton and cloth bandage. No surgical gloves, no sterile drapes and no assistants.

Many years later, I realised that our government's targets in the health sectors (especially in the family planning sector) and the budgetary restrictions created such severe constraints in most hospitals, that it pushed the healthcare personnel to step out of the safety margins. In 1968, I actually saw a Medical Officer perform vasectomies without gloves, and with a 7 O' Clock shaving razor blade as a knife! One rural surgeon from Odisha had presented a paper (I think in 1995) to show how he had to meet the tubectomy targets by performing abdominal tubectomy operations with a single pair of sterile gloves, at the home of the patient, sitting on the floor by the side of the patient who herself was lying on a mat on the floor in her sari! Only the surgeon in his working dress wore sterile gloves, while the assistant held the retractor from under the sterile drape towel! According to the *WHO Guidelines for Safe Surgery 2009*: "In the review studies published between 1950-2003, "there was no association between floor contamination dispersion and infection of the surgical wound or the rate of surgical site infections." However, no one would dream of working without gloves nowadays as it sounds crude, dirty, unhygienic, pathogenic, so on and so forth. Now even caterers wear gloves.

Coming back to the boy with the abscess, I vividly remember that scene at the neighbour's house, as if it were yesterday.

In the drawing room of the boy's home, the boy's eldest sister, who was physically strong and had a strong heart, sat cross-legged on a mat on the floor. She made the boy sit on her lap facing forward so that his knees were flexed in front of her (like sitting on a chair). She literally immobilised the boy, clamping his chest and upper arms against her chest with her right forearm. Her left hand held his legs tight. Neighbours crowded around, wide-eyed with awe; some others were peeping through the windows. My father (the doctor) sat cross-legged on the floor in front of her. There was hushed silence all around. He cleaned the skin over the abscess with spirit and then in a flash made a bold vertical incision over the abscess. That was it. The boy was unaware of what happened, until the incision was made. He suddenly screamed! Pus gushed out and filled the metal dinner plate placed under his feet. The boy's other sister fainted and collapsed to the floor. All others 'oohed' and 'aahed'. Soon the abscess was empty. My father placed some dressing over the wound and bandaged the knee. The surgery was over.

I do not remember much about the 'post-operative' medications; but I guess it would not have been much, barring some pain killing powder like aspirin, application of 'poultice' and fomentations. I am now convinced that the release of pus was the most important step in the treatment of that abscess. Gradually, the wound healed. I do not think my father got paid for the service. It was just another friendly neighbourhood help extended by a general practitioner. Recently, I met the boy, who is now an elderly man. He had nothing to show of that episode, except perhaps an inconspicuous scar!

This whole episode left a lasting impression on me. I was impressed by my father's confidence, how a bold cut with a small knife gave 'instant relief' to the boy, and so on. I too wanted to be like my father!

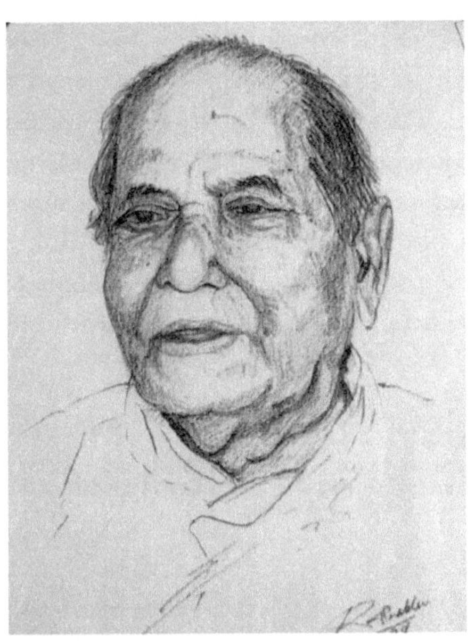

2. My Father

My father, Dr D. P. Prabhu, popularly known in Ankola as Datte-parob, the person who incised the abscess, has been a true role model for me. He has influenced my life, career and practice in many ways. Though only a licentiate medical practitioner by training, he studied and became quite adept in obstetrics also. He could extract teeth. He had an astute clinical acumen and almost all the ailments were diagnosed on clinical findings. A nephew of mine had fever that did not come down with usual treatment. My father suspected Rheumatic carditis on clinical findings and he was sent to Bombay for further investigation and treatment. He did have Rheumatic carditis and was treated in time.

He was good in many other fields too, like trees, timber and wood, grafting of plants etc. We had two mango trees, that were grafted by him. He was the first to study cement technology in Ankola, and to use it to add some extra rooms to our house; he repaired his own BMW motor-bike. A good hunter, he had shot tigers, cheetahs, bisons, wild boars, and more, with his double barrel Winchester gun. It was indeed difficult for people to gauge the full ability and potential of this man, clad in nine-yard dhoti, black coat and black cap!

My family is of agrarian lineage. But my father chose to become a doctor. It was solely because of him that I chose the medical profession over agriculture.

In our five generations that I have been able to trace, all my ancestors were landlords in a small village near Ankola, (N.K.) in the erstwhile Bombay Presidency of the British Empire! My father was the first one to break away from that agriculture. There was no school in his village. The high school was four miles away, and he would walk the distance to and fro, to come home every week end. When my father stubbornly stuck to his decision to be a doctor, the only place where he could achieve his dreams was Bombay, a really faraway place in those days of poor transportation. He had found out that a new medical college, The Topiwala National Medical College, was being started in Bombay. Overcoming all resistance and difficulties, and staying with commission agents in Bombay, who supplied commodities to our district, he got admission in the second batch for the Licentiate course of College of Physicians and Surgeons of Bombay (LCPS). Interestingly, my father in law too was a student of this college.

After getting the LCPS, he tried to set up his practice as a general practitioner in different parts of the North Kanara district, but finally settled down in Ankola, his own home town. My father was one of the two doctors looking after people in Ankola and the several miles of rural and hilly areas surrounding it. His decision to steer away from the ancestral profession saved him and his family from a future catastrophe. Our family owned a few acres of agricultural land that made us "land lords". They provided us our annual rice needs and also supplied some mangoes when in season. But my father and his brothers lost their lands following reforms in independent India that made the tiller the owner of the land. Overnight, the family of landlords became poor 'landless' lords!

As far as I can remember, our whole community was very poor during the British Raj. It affected my father's income too. Many patients could not pay at all! To be honest, we were just as poor as the rest of the community, despite being a doctor's family. Once my father had said to me that however rich a man may be, he can only eat ordinary rice or wheat like we do; he cannot eat golden rice or golden wheat just because he can afford it! I have never forgotten that.

Basic health care was totally missing in the whole district. Infrastructure as we know it now was non-existent. There was a Government Hospital in town and like now, the services there depended on the Medical Officer at the time. Most of the town went to private dispensaries. For surgeries and complicated treatments, the only place to go was Karwar, the district headquarters, where there was a surgeon in the district hospital with better facilities. But there was neither ambulance service, taxi nor convenient motor (bus) service for patients to go there. I remember a patient brought to my father from a nearby village in a hammock on two poles carried by four men (porters). Besides, poverty deterred patients from going to Karwar, which invariably meant a lot of expenses. As a result, mortality and morbidity were very high all around.

Apart from father, there was one more LCPS doing General Practice (GP), also called family practice, in the town. GP involved dispensing mixtures, powders, ointments, an occasional injection, and so on. I used to visit my father's clinic, which was called a dispensary by others, to see him at work. He would prepare cough, carminative, anti-diarrhoeal, and other mixtures for each patient individually, with separate formulae using various powders, coloured solutions and syrups from the medicine shelf. He would then stick a strip of white paper on the bottle (brought by the patient) to mark out the dosage. This practice of dispensing medicine in small bottles is the genesis of the nickname of the famous J. J. Hospital, which was also known as 'Batli Bhai' hospital when I was a student. My father's dispensary smelt of antiseptics, and other chemicals. He had to visit Bombay now and then to replenish his mixture ingredients. Later, when I was at Grant Medical College, I would bring his supplies from the shops on Princess Street or the *'dava bazaar'* in Bombay.

On one such visit, I saw a most impressive and unforgettable sight of a cataract operation on the steps of a shop. In the midst of the busy Princess Street, with cars, horse carts and hordes of people going to and fro, raising dust and noise, the patient was sitting on an ordinary office chair, head thrown back as though to see the sky. The man operating was talking loudly, *"Dekho… aaa gaya, aaa gaya, aaa gaya…,"* as he did something to the eye with his right hand, and with a forceps-like instrument in the left hand, he held up the removed cataract! I do not know if he used any anaesthesia, but the patient was quite alert. He stood up, thanked the *'dacter'*, and walked into the shop!

Most of my father's patients were our own poor workers, neighbours or relatives. So, free treatment was common! My father had to visit a number of surrounding villages too, which he usually did on a bicycle. There might have been a bus once a day to some places. But, if my father missed the return bus, he would have to spend the night in the farmer's hut! Later, he bought a motorbike. If any problem arose with the bike, he would have to fix it himself. If it did not start during a village trip, one could see a villager pushing the bike with my father seated on it! Villagers called it a 'Phat-Phat Motar'. Being the only two doctors trained in Western medicine, they both were also the last points of referral. They had to deal with all sorts of emergencies. The emergencies could be from any branch of medicine.

Our town lacked even basic life-saving medical facilities. Once our priest, who was diabetic, had a foot infection that my father could not control. The next place for treatment was Bombay, a city 800km away, to be reached by Ship Sabarmati. Many years later, when I was in medical college in the 1950s, I remember our religious guruji had a myocardial infarction (MI), while visiting Ankola. He needed oxygen, but there was not a single oxygen cylinder in the whole town, or even in the Government Hospital. In another incident, a patient recovering from typhoid suddenly developed peritonitis, probably due to a perforation of the intestine; he died of a treatable condition because his family was too poor to take him to Karwar for the life-saving surgery. A neighbour from a well-to-do family died delivering a child, due to excess blood loss! No wonder that the life expectancy in those days was about 31 years. The backwardness of the place made my father advise me to look for some other place to start my surgical practice when I returned from the UK.

My father liked obstetrics more than any other branch of medicine. He studied the subject from books and had a variety of delivery forceps, even those that were used only by qualified obstetricians. We found them useful in our practice in Shimoga. His confidence on the subject was well demonstrated to us when we started our practice. One day a woman in labour came to our nursing home (NH). I am not sure if she had had any antenatal examination at all. Dr Usha realised that it was a breech presentation (legs and bottom first delivery), which could be difficult and tricky for the untrained. We were tense, but not my father. He was there, assuring us that there is nothing to worry. He described how the delivery progresses, and how to deliver the after-coming head of the baby. His encouraging words were comforting but not convincing enough for us. Notwithstanding our indecisiveness, the labour progressed as described to us; and we had to assist in the natural process! I too had washed up to help Usha. My father was guiding us from outside the delivery room. His clear, easy to follow, step by step instructions were as though he was reading from a book, and as if he could see the baby's progress! We succeeded in delivering the baby safely.

We had alternative and native medical practitioners too. There was (and perhaps continues to be) a popular farmer who doubled as a 'bone setter' in Todur, some miles from Ankola. He treated fractures without anaesthesia, with manipulation, pastes of leaves and rustic crude splints. There was another farmer in Belambar, a suburb of Ankola, who had an herbal oil, made using a special formula, a family secret transferred from father to son, orally. Belambar oil was, and is, used for treating hemiplegia and paralysis. His oil and massages continue to be famous far and wide even now. People from faraway places like Gujarat used to come to him for treatment. Even my father used to direct some of his patients to him, seeing that it was more effective than most allopathic treatments available at that time. I sincerely believe that the ultimate goal of any doctor is to give relief to his patient; methods and medicines are only the means to an end; the system of medicine was, and is, not relevant. That became my guiding principle during my practice in Shimoga.

My father continued to give us his old wisdom and clinical guidance till the day he died, at a ripe age of 93. His interest in medicine even in his old age was very impressive.

Whenever I visited my father's dispensary, I would see him juggling medicines and syrups to prepare mixtures for patients, finishing the process by sticking a white paper on the bottle with dosage instructions; or preparing an ointment on a tile and then filling it into an empty match box; or giving an injection behind a screen! As a child, this was awe-inspiring, and made me think, "My daddy is the greatest!" I too wanted to be like him. I wanted to be a doctor too. I did not have the least idea what I was aiming for; I just wanted to emulate my idol, my father, who tried to alleviate the pain of people around us! Not having seen anything better, I had presumed that life was like this for everybody, everywhere. Frankly, it did not occur to me that healthcare could be improved and could be made available to all. So, I did not even think of improving healthcare in a broad sense. Giving relief to people around me became my goal instead. The drainage of the abscess described earlier was perhaps the first stimulus for me to pick medicine as my vocation. I felt that I too must become a doctor like my father.

3. School, Medical College, and Further

My immediate aim was to do well in high school and then get admission to a medical college. In 1947, when India became independent, I was in the Edward High School, (now Jai Hind High School) Ankola, and all the subjects were being taught in English medium. As soon as we got independence, the Government suddenly decided to change the medium of education to Kannada, our state language. The teachers were furious because all along they had been teaching their subjects in English and were not conversant with Kannada. Let alone having new textbooks, even the Kannada words for various technical subjects and topics were yet to be found! Naturally, the teachers were unhappy. Shri Ramrai Master even threw the Kannada textbook out of the window in a fit of rage! My worry was that, three years later, I would be in college, where all subjects would be taught in English only. Switching back from Kannada to English at that stage could be difficult. So, four of us who wished to go to college, met the principal (one of my favourite teachers) Shri S. P. Pikle, and made a special request to the school staff to teach us in English so that we would not face difficulties in college. They readily agreed as it was far easier for them to do so. That was a big help for our future education. I am surprised that after 70 years, this language controversy is yet to be resolved!

When the results of the Secondary School Leaving Certificate (SSLC) examinations were out (1952), I found that I have done well. First from our school. But there was no fun in it for me. Although I had done very well in the examination, five members of my family had been in a bad road accident a few days earlier (1952). All of them, including my unmarried sister, suffered severe facial injuries. Our house was like a casualty ward. Nobody was in the mood to notice my success, leave alone celebrate it.

For my college education, I had decided to go to the Karnataka College in Dharwad, which was ranked No. 1 at that time in Bombay-Karnataka. I had no problem getting admission there but the impersonal teaching methods, and having to listen to all subject lectures in English, did not please me much. Math, particularly calculus, was very difficult for me to understand. I passed the first-year exam with difficulty. The next year, we were separated into two groups – A and B. A was for mathematics students, who usually went in for engineering; and B for biology students, who usually wanted to study medicine. Obviously, I chose the B group. Now I was studying the subjects that I liked, and so I was happier too. To make sure that I would get a medical seat, I tried for extra points from extracurricular activities. During our high school days, I was in the school team that won the District Interschool Volleyball Tournament. So, I joined the volleyball team of the Karnataka College and we won a few matches too. I joined the National Cadet Corps of the 5th Bombay Battalion (NCC) and tried my best to do well in that too. I was successful in getting a rank of Cadet Corporal, of being chosen as a stick-orderly for a visiting officer Major Ukidwe, and also Certificate B of NCC Infantry. Finally, the decisive Intermediate Science Examination was over. I had done well here too, and yet could not celebrate again, because our family was abuzz with preparations for my sister's wedding (1954)!

We chose Bombay for my medical education. My cousin N. M. Prabhu was already a student there and that was an important factor. The Kasturba Medical College, Manipal, had just started and ready to admit those who could pay a huge donation to it. We could not afford the ₹5000 donation in those days. Dharwad University was in the Bombay province, and it did not have any medical college of its own. However, Bombay province had six medical colleges; three in Bombay, and one each in Pune, Ahmedabad and Baroda. So, Karnataka University students had a reservation of seats in all these Government Medical Colleges. Admission to medical colleges was strictly on merit only. It used to be said that if one passed in first class in the Intermediate Science Examination, a medical seat was assured. But gradually, though I had secured a first class we were told that there was great competition and a higher ranking would be better. I was tense. I hoped that the extracurricular activities points may help me.

At that time, I suddenly realised that I did not have a plan B in case I didn't get admitted to a medical college. I was jolted by the thought that plan B would have to be becoming a teacher in my own school! Not getting a medical seat would have been a catastrophe. When the results were announced, however, I was more than pleased; I was offered admission to all the six colleges of Bombay province. I opted for the Grant Medical College, Bombay, where my cousin was already there.

I joined college. Lectures, dissection, and other coursework began, and I soon became busy with my studies. However, towards the end of the first term in medical college, I had a major setback in my health that almost ruined my future. I had to be hospitalised and investigated by a leading physician of Bombay, Dr. M. Modi, who was an Honorary Physician in our college and hospital. Dr S. G. Desai, Registrar of the unit, found a 'murmur' in the heart. Soon their clinical conclusion was that it was a pericardial 'rub'. Next day, when the unit's Head, Dr. Modi came to our ward for rounds, the rub had 'disappeared'. But my chest X-Ray showed not only a dilated heart shadow but also a patch of tuberculosis 'infiltration' in the right lung. They did not resort to sputum examination in those days, but on the basis of clinical and radiological findings, concluded that I had tuberculosis of the lung and tuberculous pericarditis with effusion. For a while, they wanted to aspirate the pericardial effusion. But then, choosing a more conservative approach, they decided to go for a medical line of treatment and observe the effect. That was just as well. My health improved fast and the effusion disappeared soon too. But since the correct regimen of anti-TB dugs was not properly known yet, I was sent home on an 'incomplete medical regimen' that caused trouble a few years later; I had suppurating cervical tuberculous adenitis while in the UK.

My father had come to Bombay to take me home. We returned home by an overnight ship voyage that took us to Karwar. It was so enjoyable, with fresh sea breeze, cool air and the soothing rocking of the ship. At home, I recovered much faster with homely food, mother's care and Streptomycin injections administered daily by my father. A few days later, my father came and sat near me to tell me the dreadful news. Dr. Modi had advised my father that it would be unwise for me to continue with the medical studies. The rigors and the disciplines of medical education could be too strenuous for my heart, which had been battered by the tuberculous pericarditis! I knew nothing of the disease or its complications. But I was sure of only one thing – that I wanted to re-join medical college and continue my studies to become a doctor. I told this to my father and he was sympathetic enough to concede to my wishes. So, I went back to the college and luckily for me, they let me restart my studies with the batch that was admitted one year later. I lost a year of my student life but not my career.

At Grant Medical College, order of admissions was based on marks obtained in the Intermediate Science Examination. The students were grouped in batches of 20; the first 40 (Batch I and II) were the cream of the class, and the anatomy professor called them the "Arabian horses". I was surprised and fortunate enough to find myself amongst these Arabian horses of first batch! Most of the others in this batch, the real Arabian horses, the true cream, were brainy boys and girls from Bombay colleges like St. Xavier's and Elphinstone, etc. all very good in English too. I was mediocre in my studies and being in the first batch was scary of them but they were all nice and were a stimulus to me to do better.

When I re-joined the medical college a year later because of my health issue, I was fortunate enough to meet three students in my class who influenced my college life and became my intimate friends ever since. These two boys and a girl were truly brilliant students, and I was the dullard amongst them! Their company benefitted me tremendously all along and I am proud to say we (one passed away in 2020, the girl in 2024) still continue to be close friends.

One of them was Shirish Sheth, a shy, unassuming, brilliant boy with a photographic memory. He was so fond of cricket that he would hold a small transistor radio to his ear as he studied a textbook for the final MBBS examination. Now and then he would give a shout depending upon the turn of events in the match. Then at the end of it all, he would be able to recollect the textbook's contents almost verbatim. I found that scary! He became a world-renowned gynaecologist, known for his expertise in vaginal hysterectomy. He was also a very popular Professor of Obstetrics and Gynaecology at the K.E.M. Hospital and G. S. Medical College, Mumbai, and his clinical meetings or lectures were always crowded. He was also the president of the International Federation of Obstetrics and Gynaecology (FIGO).

The second one, the late Frank Sequeira, was always considered to be a scholar of our class. He became the top physician in an American oil company in Saudi Arabia, and retired to settle in Canada. If he had stayed back in Bombay, perhaps he would have become one more noted physician there.

The third, Vinodh Karani (Nee Sarwal), was very pretty, had a number of admirers, and was brilliant in her studies. She worked with Bombay's top physician and a top neuro-physician (neurologist). She later practiced as a very popular consulting physician.

In the dissection hall again one year later, I was an old hand having dissected an upper limb during the first term of my previous year. Now, my partner Pesi B. Chacha (noted Hand surgeon in Singapore, now retired) and I had to dissect the same part (forearm) that I had dissected the year before. While others were wondering what to do with the cadaver, holding kerchiefs over their noses to avoid the formalin fumes and unsure where to start, I had opened my instrument set and started the dissection. This astonished my partner Pesi, and Shirish and Frank, the other two students on our table. Then, I told them about my health story.

After completing the dissection of one part, we had to face a 'part examination' to prove our proficiency in the anatomy of that part. All the students would stand in a semi-circle facing the lecturer and he would ask questions. If you answered correctly, you stayed, otherwise you failed. Those who failed would have to do some reparative study. Our Anatomy professor, Prof. Dastur had dedicated his life to the subject. He made us study comparative anatomy by sending us to the nearby Victoria Zoo (now, Ranibagh), to study the animals there. Sometimes he would come to take the part examination of the first and second batches, which he had named the 'Arabian Horses'. Those who survived answering earlier questions, he would take them to his favourite, well-kept museum specimens to grill them further. Normally, the anatomy sections were cut horizontally, but he had some cut obliquely. The orientations of structures in them become a little more difficult. The Professor's pet student and I had survived until this stage. The oblique section stumped the pet boy, while my answer was correct. But the professor gave the credit to the pet boy; such incidents were not uncommon in the future too.

We had to pass the first MBBS examination before going for clinical training. This examination, like all future ones, was pretty hard. The examiners were from different colleges (G. M. College, G. S. M. College and the B. Y. L. Nair Medical College) and they were known to be very unfavourable to students from other colleges. We felt like sacrificial goats. I faced the examinations as best as I could, and returned home to Ankola, hoping to pass. In those days, the results would be published in the Times of India paper on a specified day. The day before the results were due, my father received a telegram from Bombay saying, "Safe Arrival." Nobody had travelled and understandably, my father was perplexed. Then, looking at the sender's name, he deduced that it was from his friend at the Times of India, and so it probably meant that I had passed my examination. Next day, we knew it was so.

4. Clinical Training

When I returned to college, all those who had passed had been divided into fresh batches of 20 each. One batch to each of the six medical and surgical units of the J. J. Group of Hospitals. All these hospitals, the college and hostels for boys and girls were situated within a huge compound spread over 44 acres in Byculla, Bombay. Everyone walked between the hospital, college and hostel.

From the smell of formalin, we switched over to that of phenyl. We equipped ourselves with a stethoscope, a percussion hammer, a little torch, white coat, etc. We attended wards until lunch time, and then there would be lectures and other demonstrations. At times we were called back to the wards in the evenings for special clinics. It took some time for me to realise the importance of this ward work. That is the place where we truly learn clinical medicine. The Unit Head and Assistant Consultants were Honorary posts; though they worked for free in the hospital, they were keen on teaching. They devoted their time sincerely to treat the patients and also to teach the students. The Registrar and even the House Surgeon tried to impart some knowledge to us during our ward attendance. Each unit had its admission day and all emergency admissions would land in its wards. So busy was this hospital that patients invariably had to be accommodated on floor beds and beds in the passages!

From my childhood I would enjoy to do things with my hands; like making a Ganapati idol for three years, arts and crafts like Deepavali lanterns, drawing and painting etc. In college, therefore I preferred the creative art of surgery more than any other subject. One day, there came a patient in the casualty department, with a 3inch long incised wound on the left forearm. The Casualty Consultant looked at it and asked me to suture it up under local anaesthesia. I infiltrated the skin edges with the local anaesthetic and put around four or five skin sutures. The wound edge approximation and the end results were so neat that the Casualty Consultant jokingly asked me to take up a surgical career. I am not sure if that remark decided my future at all, but it could have influenced me subconsciously. Practical work by hands appealed to me more than theoretical problem-solving.

Our first surgical term was in the unit headed by Dr H Doctor, a capable surgeon in those days. We were in the gallery of the operation theatre when Dr Doctor started the abdominal surgery. He took a bold incision in the upper abdomen and blood started to spurt out of the wound. I felt faint at this sight and had to sit down, but this never happened again. Later, in Shimoga, where we set up our surgical nursing home, my nephews and nieces who aspired to become doctors, wanted to see me perform a surgery in Shimoga. Most of them fainted at the sight of the blood. One of them felt very embarrassed. But later, she told us that in her medical college, she was proud to have been the only one still on her feet while all her colleagues were flat on the floor at the sight of blood!

Then we shifted to medical wards. During these clinical (wards) terms, we were taught clinical medicine to find out the pathology inside the body of a patient with our own five senses – eyes, hands, smell, ears and so on, along with aids like the stethoscope and percussion hammer. Our old Ayurveda thousands of years ago, had "trividha" (three types) "Ashtavidha" (eight ways of) and "Dasha-vidha Pareeksha"(ten types) of examinations that were far superior! Now, we have advanced with wonderful gadgets like sonography, radiology, CT scan and MRI to detect the same.

Finally, we had an obstetrics term when each of us had to conduct or assist in ten normal deliveries. If any patient needed Caesarean section delivery (not very common in those days), the big bell in the Bai Motlibai Obstetric Hospital would be rung for all to hear in the campus, to invite anyone interested in watching it. Nowadays, that operation is a commonplace event!

In the extracurricular fields, my love for NCC made me join the newly-started Naval Medical Unit. This gave me an opportunity to represent the Bombay University NCC at the National Youth Festival in Delhi, get a B and a C Certificate from Naval NCC, and also to become a Cadet Captain (Naval). I was surprised to learn that there are 21 different uniforms for Naval men! We were taken to Lonavala Naval base and to Visakhapatnam for our two annual training camps, and to the local Ashvini Naval Hospital at Colaba, which kindled a slight interest in me to consider a career in the Navy. But the regimentation and the drill put me off.

Final MBBS examination was a frightful experience just like the other examinations, where examiners tried to pull down the candidates from other medical colleges. I was very diffident. Somehow, the examination was over and I was relieved to know that I had passed.

Ours was the second (or third) batch to be put through the newly-introduced year-long internship training. It was not yet fully structured and so there was less of training and more of manual labour like taking patients from one place to another, taking blood samples to labs, collecting the lab reports, getting the X-rays, pre-operation scrubbing of patients, and so on. Community Medicine term for three months was a virtual holiday, six weeks of Rural Medicine in Palghar was used for learning to play bridge, visiting the sea side for fish fry, and such fun. The Medical Officer was not interested in us except for one night when we all went out to collect blood samples for Malaria. Urban Term of six weeks was no better. We visited a hotel in Dadar, which was selected by the Health Department. The hotel obeyed all health precautions. Rest of the days were to ourselves!

Now I was fully qualified and got the degree of M.B.B.S.

As I said before, I liked surgery more than any other branch of medicine available in those days. But I did not make the required grade to get admission for post graduate course in surgery. Only the top students would apply for and get a seat for the MS course. Most of them also got a Registrar post and a stipend. I could not compete with them. Post-graduation in India, without the stipend, would have been economically non-viable for me. That was the time when there was a great demand for Indian doctors in the USA and UK. Many of my classmates appeared for the Educational Commission for Foreign Medical Graduates (ECFMG) examination and chose to go to the USA and settle there. There were no entry tests to go to the UK. My cousin had gone to the UK and by now had passed the Fellowship of the Royal College of Surgeons (FRCS) exam. Our medical education at the time was more of British methods and techniques and I liked the conservative approach of the British to each problem. Besides, my cousin was already in the UK. So, I chose to go to the UK to earn, learn and aim for the Fellowship in surgery.

While preparing for this trip to the UK, I completed two 'house jobs' of six months each – one of them being surgical. The unit head was Dr R. A. Irani, with Dr Rasik Patel as his assistant, Dr. Hakim, who was my classmate the previous year, was the registrar. Like all units, there was so much to do and learn, that I never managed to finish it all in time. Once a week on an 'admission' (emergency) day, House surgeon had to write down notes of all admitted patients, do their urine and blood examinations himself, get other investigations if any needed, before the ward rounds the next day. Then prepare those that needed surgery by scrubbing their operation area and then go to the O. T. to assist. This was too strenuous and most houses surgeons faked the time consuming and unnecessary, investigations. Our college had many Indian students from Africa. They would work as supernumerary (without any stipend) house surgeons just to get registration with the Indian Medical Council (IMC) before returning to Africa. Second House surgeon (supernumerary) in our unit was one such doctor. I was asked to look after the male ward, and the supernumerary house surgeon was to work in the female ward. But the work in the female ward used to be perpetually incomplete, with dressings not done, incomplete notes and such problems, and our Registrar, Dr Hakim would quietly come to me and request me to cover him up! At the end of the day, I used to be dead tired.

J. J. Hospital was situated in a high crime area; violence, murders and stabbings were common. During one of our nights of emergency duty, a patient came with a knife stuck in his chest. He was wheeled to the OT directly and Dr Patel opened his chest to find the knife blade in the left ventricle of the heart. He removed the knife and the blood spurted all over. Dr Patel put his thumb into the hole in the heart to stop the blood loss, was not sure what to do; he looked at our registrar Dr Hakim, and asked us all in Gujarati, "Ave shu karoo? (What shall we do now?)" All were silent. So, he took Size 2 Chromic Catgut and put a figure-of-eight suture around the hole and tied it. Talk of presence of mind and innovation! The bleeding stopped. He then closed the chest and transferred the patient to the thoracic unit the next day. This was a lesson to me showing how a surgeon has to think outside the box as they say, to tide over a life threatening crisis. At the end of the six months of the job, Dr. Hakim was generous to permit me to operate on one hydrocele patient!

These jobs helped me get my hands wet with blood and introduced me to the basic surgical procedures. They also helped in registering with the General Medical Council (GMC) of the UK. J. J. Group of Hospital jobs were recognised by the General Medical

Council for registration. That was also the time when a passport was good enough to get entry into the UK; visas were not started yet.

So, I started getting ready to go to the UK. While applying for a passport, we realised my date of birth did not have documentary evidence; we did not have a birth registry in those days in Ankola. My father had to sign an affidavit under oath, confirming my date of birth. The next challenge was travel. Air travel was out of my reach. Some classmates of mine and other friends formed a group to travel by sea, on P&O liner SS Strathmore. We left on 12th of February 1962. The cheapest berths (90 pounds sterling each) were in the innermost bowels of the ship but we were in a group and that did not matter. It took 15 days to reach London from Bombay. But the time was well worth it, as it familiarised us with British customs and practices, use of knife and fork and food choices, the old weather, table etiquette, and so on. Some of us were bold enough to spend five pounds sterling, out of 13 pounds cash generously permitted by the Govt. of India, for a land trip to the Pyramids of Giza in Cairo. It was the time of Algerian war too! Passing through the Mediterranean was over, but the Bay of Biscay tossed the ship so much that all of us were severely sea sick. Finally, on a very cold 27th of February morning, we arrived at the Tilbury docks on the famous river Thames. We took a boat train to the Victoria Station in London. I do not recall any one checking our passports even, for our entry into the UK. My friend M. K. Shanbhag was waiting at the Victoria station and I went with him to his flat at Cromwell crescent, in Earls Court. That was my transit place till I found a job.

5. Training in the UK

Registration with the G.M.C. was necessary to get a job in any National Health Service Hospital; I could get only 'temporary registration' since I had done only one recognised house job in India. After I finished another six months in NHS hospital, I would qualify for the permanent registration. I also had to have a Medical Insurance. By now hospital jobs were difficult to get, due to the sudden influx of immigrant doctors. To get a job, most of the recommendations by our Indian consultants and the certificates from Mumbai were worthless; a word from a person to them was more effective. My cousin had worked at the North Staffordshire Royal Infirmary in Stoke-on-Trent and on his recommendation, I got my first surgical house job there.

But, before I start talking about my experiences in the UK, and the people I met there, I must share with you that it is customary in the UK to address surgeons as Mister, Miss, Mrs or Ms. While in the rest of the world, all medical practitioners including physicians and surgeons are addressed as Doctor (Dr.), in the United Kingdom, all fellows of a Royal College of Surgeons (something like MS Surgery in India) are addressed as Mr, Miss, Mrs or Ms, and these titles are considered to be of a higher status than Dr.

So, coming back to my first surgical house job, the surgeon, Mr Grocott the consultant, was a General Surgeon but was also trained as a Plastic Surgeon by the Father of Modern Plastic Surgery, Sir Harold Gillis. So, Mr G managed a burns unit in addition to the general surgeries and did many corrective procedures like cleft lips, and cleft palates, treatment of maxillofacial injuries, breast reductions and so on. He stressed and taught me that in a road traffic accident injury, removing all the grit and dirt from every abrasion and wound is more important than the cosmetic perfections. He even used stiff nail brush to dislodge the grit even if lead to profuse bleeding! Once healed, the embedded grit look like tattoo marks and are very difficult to remove. I decided to learn as much as possible from him. He rarely used skin markings even for cleft lips, except for breast reductions in private wards, applied simple interrupted skin sutures, and used plain cotton thread for skin sutures. The results were wonderful, showing that technique is more important than suture material.

It was difficult to adjust to British food and tastes. A significant number of the other residential doctors were also Indian. So, every Sunday there would be Indian-style cooking by the Indian doctors, the quintessential '*dal-bhaat*'. That pleased the semi-starved Indian doctors to some extent. My cousin had introduced me to Dr Bose, an anaesthetist, as a local guardian. He was very friendly and advised me on many aspects of life there. He also insisted that I learn to eat cheese daily. But the bland British dishes and cheeses did not appeal very much to me then. However, by the time I completed my stay in the UK, I had developed a liking for the very same bland British dishes and developed a taste for the salty cheeses like Roquefort. Life in the UK was far better than that in India. Working hours were busy but off-duty time was my own. Accommodation, food and laundry were free and the salary though meagre by present standards, was all saved and credited to the bank every month. Fee for signing a death certificate was a Pound sterling, enough to pay for sundry personal petty expenses! I hoped to save enough money to do a refresher course in the Royal College of Surgeons, London before appearing for the primary FRCS examination.

All was going well, when tuberculosis raised its head again. I had cervical adenitis and fever. Surprisingly the gland biopsy result was 'negative' and so I continued my job and took up the next one too – a house job in the very busy Orthopaedic department of the same hospital. The department had three consultants; one of them was Mr Wainwright, who had devised his own 'pin and plate' for a femoral neck fracture. Fracture of the neck of the femur was treated as a semi emergency case; internal fixation was performed as a priority. This saved longer hospitalisation and the morbidity thereby. The hospital was in a colliery district and accidents there and the road accidents kept our department very busy. I learnt a lot of orthopaedics in these six months. I even had to perform a lumber puncture for a myelography!

Of the three consultants in this Orthopaedic unit, two were very academic and loved by the junior staff. The third, Mr M, though not very popular with the junior doctors, was the most successful orthopaedist in town. Reportedly, he had a huge private practice, mostly of old patients. He wore a Saville Row suit, and used to come in a Bentley car (next only to Rolls Royce in quality, cost and opulence). In his out-patient clinic, he was known to greet his patients in person cheerfully. "How is our darling today?" he would say to an old lady in a wheelchair. He was also known for giving intra-articular cortisone for chronic badly-arthritic knee joints. The old girl would then get up from her wheelchair and walk 'painlessly' to her car, cooing all the while, "Oh, isn't he a lovely man!" Obviously, M's success could be attributed to his satisfied patients – a lesson for me to take home.

There was a clinical meeting for the junior doctors. Speaker was Dr. Kerr a physician with FRCP. It is said that a Fellowship of Royal College of Physicians is an honorary Diploma given to distinguished physicians. Dr. Kerr showed his brilliance in his presentation. He was given only a chest X-Ray of a patient and was asked to discuss the differential diagnosis from it. History of the patient, physical findings, other lab investigations were not given. He discussed each finding on the X-Ray in such masterly manner that he concluded on the correct diagnosis of an uncommon lung condition. Everyone cheered him loudly.

After this job, I registered for a refresher course by the Royal College of Surgeons, London. The earnings of the last one year were just about enough to pay for the course, with accommodation in the RCS hostel in Lincoln's Inn Fields, and the examination fee.

When I started the refresher course, I had also paid for accommodation in the RCS hostel. The incompletely-treated tuberculosis raised its head yet again and this time it was a proper 'cold abscess' on my neck. I went to the nearby Charing Cross Hospital where Dr Plummer admitted me and had the abscess drained and curetted. Dr. Plummer's ward round was very interesting. There were only 5-6 students in the batch (we were 20 in each batch back home). Dr. P knew each student by his name. He would involve each student in the discussion. This time there was no doubt that it was tuberculous adenitis. Realising that I am attending the refresher FRCS course, and that I did not have the prescribed number of Streptomycin injection after the pericarditis, he advised that I take the balance number of Streptomycin injections at home every day along with two other medications – para-amino salicylic acid (PAS) and isoniazid (INH). These along with syringes, needles etc. were supplied by the N.H.S. free of cost. A Dr Pillai, who also was doing the course with me, helped me with the injections, and I completed that course of injections and drugs. The wound healed but I missed a lot of lectures. So, instead of appearing for the primary FRCS examination in London, I decided to appear in Dublin, Ireland, where the examination was about a month later. Dr Pillai, two others and I went to Dublin a week before the examination and stayed as paying guests.

The examination was in a few days' time. On one weekend, our host, Mrs. McLaughlin, promised that we would have Chicken

Biryani on Sunday. We were thrilled and eagerly waited for the Sunday. Come Sunday, we could not believe our eyes when she served us cooked rice mixed with some pieces of chicken, tomato ketchup and *sultanas*. That was her biryani!

The Anatomy and Physiology taught in our refresher course was almost similar to what we learnt in first year MBBS in Grant Medical College. Dr Sethna, the Assistant Professor of Anatomy there, was a teacher in the J. J. School of Arts too. He taught us anatomy of the abdomen with beautiful diagrams of transverse sections, one each going through thoracic 12th to Lumbar 5th vertebrae. With these sections, he explained the anatomy of all the abdominal organs, vessels, nerves, and so on. As he drew these sections on the black board, with different coloured chalks for different tissues, I copied them in my notebook with similar coloured pencils. With the drawings of these six sections, one could describe anatomy of any abdominal organ or nerve structure very clearly. After my first MBBS examination, this notebook just disappeared from my room. Reportedly, it did rounds in the ladies' hostel. Finally, it mysteriously reappeared when I was doing a house surgeon job. I was happy to find it. When I appeared for the Primary FRCS examination in Dublin, there were three questions in the anatomy paper from this thin notebook alone! I happily answered those with the colourful drawings of these sections from this notebook! Oral examinations, viva-voce as some call it, were in the afternoon. We went into a pub for some light snacks. My friends ordered a pint of beer each, but I hesitated. I asked for a cup of coffee. "We don't have coffee here, sir," the barman said. Then he stopped and said, "Oh yes, I can give you fresh Irish coffee if you like." Innocently, I said yes. After a long time, he came with a small glass of dark liquid, which looked somewhat like coffee decoction. No milk. I said, "My bad luck," and sipped it. It smelt strongly of whiskey! I asked him what it was, and he said that Irish coffee is coffee in Irish whiskey! I did not drink any of it and went for our examination. In the evening, we learnt that only I had passed, but again, there was no cheer as the other three that came with me had failed!

Now I took up a Casualty Officer (Senior House Officer) job in Walsall, near Birmingham. I was expected to assist ENT, Orthopaedics and ophthalmology wards too; a duty I could not fulfil properly. After duty hours, and when I had free time, I would attend the orthopaedic out-patient department attached to the casualty department. In the evenings, I utilised my free time to learn motor driving from the British School of Motoring at one pound per hour of hands-on teaching. Beginner, according to the BSM, needs a minimum of ten lessons (ten hours). They said the driving tests are very tough; not more than 20 percent pass at the first attempt. I learnt to drive in a Herald car that had clear visibility all round and was light too. All my lessons were in the evenings of those cold dark winter days. Driving during daytime appeared to be 'a piece of cake' as they say. With some luck I passed the examination at the first attempt, which surprised my colleagues. But I did not have a vehicle yet.

There was news of a war between India and Pakistan. Patriotism of Indian doctors, and also of Pakistani doctors, made them talk of the 'duty to help the country' by collecting funds, and such activities. But after a few days all that enthusiasm fizzled out! Soon it was time to celebrate Christmas and the New year. My colleague in the casualty department, a Dr Mike Turner was a married man. He said that they always have a 'do' in their house to greet the New Year and that I must join him. When I actually went to his house across the street from the hospital, the only drink available and served was scotch whiskey! Dr Turner would not take a No and I had to accept neat whisky in a glass. This was my first experience with whiskey. I tried to sip the first serving slowly; Dr Turner came and lifted the glass 'bottom up' and the whole of it went down my throat. I started seeing two lights, and if I closed my eyes the objects would go round in circles. I realised that I couldn't take any more and requested Dr Turner to let me go to my room. As I left his house and stepped outside, the cold air struck my face and brought back sobriety. I could safely reach my bed and sleep, as all others were greeting the New Year.

As I finished the Casualty job, and while waiting for the next job, I purchased a used Morris Minor car for 200 pounds. I got a job in Ryhope General Hospital near Sunderland in North East UK. With M.K.Shanbhag with me, I drove from London to Ryhope in my new possession the Morris Minor! I must point out that the highways were not crowded like now and it was pre motorways days. The Ryhope hospital was in sheds constructed during the war time, but had all the amenities, comfortable and neat. It was said that during the war the hospitals were kept going with the help of Indian junior doctors. In gratitude for their service, they continued employing Indian doctors, by preference, for most of their junior jobs. When I joined too there were many Indian doctors in the doctors' quarters. So much so that the kitchen staff had learnt to cook Indian dishes and even tasty chicken curry and *chapatis* on occasions.

There were two surgeons; Mr Sanford and Mr Kempsey. Mr Sanford was FRCS and MRCP (Membership of the Royal Colleges of Physicians – a post-graduate qualification in the UK). He was there during the war and had to work despite great cuts in the hospital budgets. When catgut was not available during the war, he used ordinary threads for all types of sutures including sub-cutaneous bleeders, intra-abdominal ligatures, intestinal anastomosis other than mucosal anastomoses and skin sutures. He continued that practice during peacetime too; he said, "If it can work during war time, it can work during peace too. Besides it saves a lot of precious hospital funds." I admired his spirit to reduce the cost of treatment. There would be an occasional stitch abscess in the follow-up clinic. He would just probe the wound and find the offending thread suture and remove it; the wound would then heal. I realised that this outlook and principle suited my future practice in India; I too continued most of his practices on return to India (except for the subcutaneous ties) and there were no occasions to regret! Mr Sanford believed that the floor dust causes wound infections. So he sprinkled water on the O.T. floor and outside; the wheels of the stretcher that wheeled a patient to the O.T. went through a trough of antiseptic solution. As written before. he did not believe in sterilising operation skin area with tincture iodine or Betadine; he called it 'black magic'. Instead, he made the patient take a bath with Phiso-Hexidine soap the previous night. Next day, on the operation table, he would expose the part to be operated upon and put the incision without further 'painting'. The other surgeon, Mr Kempsey was FRCS too, a conservative and academic surgeon. He used skin paints. The ward was common for both patients, and the ward sister kept a register of wound infections meticulously. Interestingly, the incidence of wound infection, and the bacterial flora in their patients, was almost the same!

Ryhope is a colliery area. I organised a trip for some of us doctors, to one of the coal mines. Similarly, we visited a brewery too to see the huge vats, and distillation units.

One year in Ryhope gave me a lot of surgical experience and confidence. I was permitted to perform many surgeries independently. Mr Kempsey was a specialist in varicose vein surgeries. He used to have long lists of patients waiting for surgery. So he took me to a hospital in the next town, where he operated, and made me perform varicose vein surgeries as he saw patients in his out-patient department. The Senior Registrar from Sunderland who visited our hospital let me perform gastric resections also.

It was time for me to appear for the final FRCS examination. Again, with my meagre savings, I attended a refresher course by the Royal College of Surgeons of Edinburgh in Scotland which was near to Ryhope, and then appeared for the examination. Happily, I passed. Once again, the joy was short lived; my very close friend who was appearing for the primary FRCS examination developed cold feet and did not write the papers at all. He was an excellent surgeon, but not much could be done without the vital letters after his name. He opted for general practice, married, settled down, and died in the Nottingham area as a very popular and successful general practitioner.

Now, I was looking for a registrar job. Opportunity came when there was a call for applications for the post of Residential Surgical Officer (RSO) in the Eastbourne group of hospitals, down south near Brighton. Whenever there were British doctors amongst the interview candidates, we, the non-British candidates were prepared to face disappointments. That was no different from what happens in Indian colleges and hospitals. I was prepared to be disappointed. Consultant Mr Peter Smith from Eastbourne hospital asked me why I wanted this particular job. I innocently blurted out the truth that I wanted to get some more experience before I went back to India. My intention of going back caught his attention, as he explained some days later. Eastbourne Hospital was affiliated to the King's College of London and surgical registrars from there got posted to Eastbourne by rotation. Such registrars lost their place on the promotion ladder for the senior registrar jobs. The senior registrar job is essential for a consultant job next. Mr Smith did not wish to take away the good prospects of a British registrar. So, I got the job. This was the job that made me whatever I was, or am, as a surgeon. So much encouragement, so much practical experience and guidance, that it gave me confidence to face all the difficulties to settle as a surgeon in a small town.

As RSO I had to work for four general surgeons, an orthopaedician, a urologist, two obstetrics and gynaecology units, two ophthalmologists, an ENT doctor and casualty! I could not honestly serve them all; but I devoted more time to surgery, casualty, orthopaedics and urology. There were four house surgeons for the four units and I was the RSO for them. The House surgeons had to attend to emergency "calls" from other consultant's wards too except for Obg&Gynae. However, being the only RSO for four units, I was required to be on duty continuously from Monday to Friday every week and in addition from Friday morning to Monday evening once in four weeks for emergencies. But this hard work made me gain a lot of confidence and experience. Mr Smith said he was happy that I wished to serve in my own country. He said that health care in India was poor (now, the Lancet Commission on Global Health has shown that 32.9 percent of all deaths in the poorest regions of the world were lost from conditions needing surgical care). Infrastructure of health care also being poor, he said that one may need to resort to 'jungle surgery'.

Jungle Surgery is a term to describe an old-fashioned surgery, which depends more on clinical approach, and less on investigations. It includes simpler procedures from other surgical branches also, and simplifies the current procedures. He took upon himself the job to train me for that jungle surgery. That appealed to me and I concentrated more on that type of surgery. It was just as well.

In the UK, most of us learnt basics of cooking for our own survival. I too had learnt some dishes. So, one day, I invited our outgoing consultant Mr and Mrs Estcourt for dinner in our doctors' quarters; I prepared for him and his wife some chicken curry of Indian recipe, rice and fried fish-mackerel! They both relished and enjoyed the meal so much that, in return, they invited me to their house to eat a typical British meal! How wonderful and generous of them. The nice fallout of this get-together was that, Mrs Estcourt was shocked by the shabby rooms, furniture and decor of our doctors' quarters. She was a member of a society called Friends of the Hospital, or something like that. She promptly saw to it that our quarters were provided with fitted floor carpets, new furniture, new curtains, and more. The chicken curry worked wonders. Mr and Mrs Smith too enjoyed my cooking very much.

Mr Smith was one of the four surgeons I was to work with. Three others, including Mr Estcourt, were GP surgeons; a post that was reportedly created to fill up the shortage of general surgeons soon after the start of the NHS. They were actually general practitioners, who were trained in surgery over a short time. If they could pass the FRCS examination from Edinburgh or one of the other colleges, they could work as part-time consultant surgeons in the hospital. We had a GP anaesthetist too. Mr Smith was the only proper FRCS (England), full-time surgeon there at the time. He took me under his wings and never missed a chance to show me how the case in hand would be treated in 'jungle surgery'. Clinical diagnosis without too many investigations was his forte.

Estbourne hospitals were in a part of the UK that was a favourite of the retiring elderlies. Breast cancer was one of the common pathologies to deal with. Mr Smith would diagnose a lump clinically in the out-patient department as malignant and admit the lady immediately, as a 'semi-emergency' overriding the waiting list. With only basic lab tests and health check-up, she would be taken up for surgery (mastectomy), in the next operation list, again as a semi-emergency! Once I asked him how he could be so sure of the diagnosis of cancer without a biopsy. Those were the days before sonography, needle biopsy etc. Mr Smith looked at me and smiled. He said that, in the last many years, his diagnosis was wrong only twice! That shows how good his clinical acumen was. His surgical techniques too were very neat. In breast surgery, he applied artery forceps to a vessel before dividing and ligated each bleeder individually; no cautery. We hardly ever saw any complications. He did not resort to lab tests like electrolyte estimation for the first two postoperative days. He rarely asked for culture sensitivity tests except in extreme cases. Simple basic antibiotics and early ambulation were the order of the day. On the day sutures were removed, he would tell the patient with a smile, "Now, you may go home, have a scratch, have a bath and a smoke…!" Mr Smith's way of surgery and his guidance were very apt for my future practice in India.

I had been warned of Mr Smith's dislike for Indians. But I did not find any such thing; in fact, he was more friendly with me than any other consultant I had worked for until now! When I rang him up about an emergency surgery that needed to be done, he would ask me if I felt confident to handle it. If yes, he would let me carry on. In the early days he would quietly visit the operation theatre without letting me know, and look over my shoulder. If all was well, he would just slip away as quietly, and no one would tell me that he had visited.

During one of such visits of his, I was performing an emergency operation on a patient with intestinal obstruction with a huge volvulus of the large intestine. I had not seen a volvulus until then. In a volvulus the intestinal loop twists on itself so that the contents cannot go forwards. Text books advise performing colostomy to relieve the obstruction as a first stage and then later, perform the excision of the redundant loop. I was not aware of all that. I felt that if I excised the offending loop everything would be alright. I did exactly that and re-joined the remaining two ends of the gut. There was no spillage of the contents and the peritoneum did not get soiled either. Patient recovered well and soon. I did not know that Mr Smith had been watching the operation all along! Next day he asked me about the emergency surgery and then said he too would have done the same thing as I did, though the books advised differently. I felt relieved.

Then one day he complimented me for having "a good pair of hands" and told me about his supervision. He said he was satisfied enough to let me do surgeries independently by myself. That was the best certificate I could get during my training; good enough to give me courage to start my surgical carrier after returning home! Being good and popular with the G.P.s of the area, Mr Smith always had a long waiting list of common surgeries. Soon he started a special Wednesday afternoon parallel session of surgeries by me in the adjacent OT, to reduce his waiting list. When we both finished in the evening, he would wait for me and take me to the local 'Tallyho' pub across the road for a glass of lager with lime. We truly got on well.

One day early in this job, a patient with abdominal pain was admitted and the British house surgeon could not come a definite diagnosis. She informed me about the patient and said she felt we could wait till the next morning and re-examine. She felt her conclusion was correct. As was my habit I went to see and examine the patient for myself. All the symptoms pointed to a possible appendicular problem but abdominal examination was inconclusive. I did a per rectal examination (a mandatory part of every abdominal examination). Patient suddenly jumped with pain deep in his pelvis; a ha, a pelvic appendicitis! I performed the emergency surgery and removed infected appendix. House surgeon was humble, impressed and complimented me.

Of the other three GP Consultants, one was about to retire- Mr. Estcourt, and after some time a new, and young, consultant came in. The new surgeon was good and academically well-qualified. The other two were very messy surgeons. One of them would give spinal anaesthesia himself before he did prostatectomies though there was a qualified G.P. anaesthetist at the head end. He did not want me in the O.T. on his days! The remaining one also operated in a haphazard manner. I decided that these two were showing me how not to perform surgeries.

Working with an orthopaedic surgeon and being in charge of the casualty (emergency) department gave me additional experience in the field of trauma surgery and orthopaedics. I even got an opportunity to perform a hip replacement (Austen Moore) surgery!

By now I had started liking western classical music, especially orchestras rendering opuses of Beethoven, Motzart, etc. ballet music etc. I even assembled a turn-table for L.P. discs, two speakers and amplifier. I brought the whole set back with me to India but hectic schedule of our nursing home practice hardly spared time to use those.

I felt that having come so far to the UK, I needed to visit some parts of Europe at least. So, with my friend Dr Subhash Sardesai, who had a new Ford car, we planned a 'camping' tour of Europe because that was the cheapest way of touring. Every tourist place in Europe has camping areas, each with basic facilities and even power and water supply, utilities stores etc. We bought the basic camping kit consisting of things like a tent, small gas stove and saucepans, ground sheets and sleeping bags, and had a wonderful, though tiring, 15 days in Europe. We would have breakfast in our tent and then hit the road. Lunch and dinner would be outside. We covered France, Belgium, Lichtenstein, Germany, Austria, Italy, Rome and Switzerland; we had to have visas for each of these countries. One night in Germany, it rained heavily and we had to run in search of hotel accommodation. Looking at two gentlemen seeking accommodation, two hotels refused us entry, probably thinking that we were gay! We had to find some other hotel. Our last lap was in Paris. But we were so tired that we were not in a mood to see any part of Paris fully nor even the famous Notre Dame cathedral! We returned a day earlier than planned.

While in Eastbourne, I appeared for the final FRCS examination in London, but did not succeed. Mr Smith was upset. "How can they fail you!" he said. He said he would come the next time and sit beside the examiner. But next time, the need did not arise. During the oral examination, the examiner asked me how I would sterilise the skin over an operation site. I replied in honesty the practice of Ryhope hospital and he was humble enough to accept it. The examiner said that in his hospital they used tincture iodine. That was all. I admired the examiner who respected and accepted Mr. Sanford's 'no skin paints' practice. I had passed the exams (1967). I was thrilled, and this time there was nothing to stop my celebration. I went to the Cromwell Crescent flat with a bottle of champagne to celebrate with the Shanbhags. The first taste of champagne was not nice; lager with lime any day!

Having gotten that which I had come to get, it was time to go home to India. Being away from home for over five years had made me very home sick! In the final year of my stay in the UK, I started buying and collecting instruments and articles that would be useful for my practice in India. I spent most of my meagre savings in the UK to buy a set of general surgery instruments, especially tungsten carbide tipped scissors, fine dissection scissors, very fine artery forceps, a sigmoidoscope, a good cystoscope set, and a ward suction unit (that served me for forty years or so) etc. OT sisters in the UK showed me some used instruments and tray boilers that were considered old and 'not usable'. I could buy them all at scrap value; they were very handy in my practice here in India for many years. By then, Indian instrument manufacturers also had improved and I bought my remaining requirements from them. In addition to the instruments and gadgets, I had also bought some household appliances like a refrigerator and a small oven. All that had to be transported by ship.

I had stayed in the UK for aboutfive and a half years continuously! I was very, very keen on going back to my home.

6. Back in India: Job or Private Practice?

Finally, I came home to India in September of 1967. I bought an air ticket just to have the experience of air travel. Once again racism was very obvious; crew on the plane devoted all their time for white skinned passengers and ignored likes of me!

I had not decided what to do next – find a job, or start my own practice. If I were to start a private practice, where shall it be? Every place had disadvantages and lacked infrastructure for a surgical practice. My hometown was too small for a surgical practice; there was absolutely nothing to support a surgical nursing home. While waiting for this decision, I found a job as Senior Lecturer of Surgery in a new, upcoming, private 'donation' medical college. This was the time I got married too – in the age-old style of 'arranged marriage'. It was nice to have a companion at home.

I had never done any teaching before, but it did appeal to me enough to make me think of making a career of it. Students too responded favourably to me. I treated students with respect and affection. But probably because I did not belong to their community, I was a misfit in that college. I was targeted and harassed for petty things. People speak of victimisation of Indian doctors in the NHS hospitals of the UK, but I am sure it could never be as bad as what

I went through during this job in India. After about one and a half years, I could not take it anymore and became so angry that I resigned from my post in the college with immediate effect without any plans for my future. I was married by now, and my wife and father were surprised at the turn of events.

I was in contact with my mentor and friend Mr Smith in the UK during all this time. He could appreciate my frustration and unhappiness. He on his own decided to create a Casualty Consultant job in the hospital where I had worked before. He offered it to me if I ever decided to return to the UK. It was a good offer, a good life in the UK. I was tempted to accept the offer. After discussing this with my family I started packing my bags to return to the UK. My father was disappointed; he made a last appeal. Having come to India with all the instruments, equipment, and other preparations to start a nursing home practice, why not give it a try for at least a year to see how things turn out, he said. My earlier inner resolve to work in my own country and now my father's appeal won over and I cancelled our plan of returning to the UK. I decided to start a nursing home practice here in India itself, come what may. Around ten years later (1980), when I happened to be in the UK, Mr Smith showed me the new District General Hospital and the job that was meant for me – a Casualty Consultant post. Of course, it was comfortable and nice but by that time I had a good practice here in Shimoga, had moved to a purpose-built nursing home and had settled well too. Life in India and the practice of jungle surgery was far superior to life in the UK doing casualty work.

Once I decided to stay in India, the next question was where to setup my practice. My father had already ruled out our hometown. Some of my friends were keen that I go to Shimoga as it did not have any surgeons in the private sector. The town had a huge government McGann hospital, considered to be the best district hospital in the whole state of Karnataka outside of Bangalore! There were surgeons, orthopaedists, obstetricians and gynaecologists, ENT specialists, ophthalmologists, and so on. Surprisingly, such a big hospital did not have a qualified anaesthetist, radiologist, pathologist or a pathology lab. The rich people of Shimoga went to Bangalore (275 km) for treatment. The middle class and the poor did not have a choice but would be happy to be treated in a private nursing home. The hospital had all the bad practices that were seen in other government hospitals. Mothers who delivered had to pay the staff to see the face of their own baby – more if it happened to be a boy. You had to pay a fee to the anaesthetist for the pre-operation check. Doctors would do the surgery only if you deposited the prescribed amount beforehand, and on top of all this, patients were diverted to private nursing homes where the same physician would go to treat. There was a Government Nursing School training for Ancillary Nursing Midwives (ANM) also; but all the students had to join government service after qualification. When I started my practice in Shimoga, I offered my free services to the patients in that hospital. The Health Minister first welcomed the idea but later, for some unknown reason, he declined.

We visited the town of Shimoga to see for ourselves my chances to set up a private surgical practice. Some important people gave encouraging responses to my desire to start a surgical practice in Shimoga. So, I decided to try my luck there. The only place we could rent for our nursing home was an old house, which was identified by many as a haunted house or 'bhoot bangla'. I was told that many occupants had failed in their trade there and so I should avoid it too. But we were desperate and leased it for five years. We actually did well in that house.

The next big challenge was setting up and equipping the nursing home. There were no books on starting of a nursing home, furnishing one, or equipping it. We had to visit a friend's nursing home, imagine the requirements and then make enquiries about the suppliers. I wondered how important were 'hospital' beds that give multiple positions, tilts etc. other special furniture and fixtures in providing good healthcare. They were all relatively costly. Our finances could not afford such furniture. I recalled that many of the newly-started NHS hospitals in the UK had old-fashioned bed steads only; they were not standard hospital beds. Obviously, we too had to compromise on all our modern requirements. The layout of the building too was for a residential house and so we had to re-orient it to the needs of a nursing home. A bedroom of about 8x10 ft. became an OT, the kitchen area became the Delivery Room, the hall transformed into a ward, a couple of single rooms, and a couple of consultation rooms. We bought cheap iron or steel household bedsteads (cots), and got some other furniture assembled in the local workshops. We used wooden blocks to raise the head-end or foot-end of the bed whenever needed. We did not think more sophisticated beds were required for the type of surgeries performed in our nursing home at the time.

Just to show how much talent was available locally, one workshop owner, an engineer by training, was so good that he created in his workshop an instrument trolley with castors, a stretcher- trolley, a simple wheelchair, some drip stands and even Thomas' splints in adult and child sizes. We used them all till we closed our 45 years of practice! Our operation table was an old fixed-height steel table that belonged to my father-in-law (LCPS) who loved performing minor surgeries on it. It could also give lithotomy, head down positions. I used this table for the next 15-16 years. Then we bought a 'hydraulic' operation table just to be 'modern' or 'updated'. I realised then that the extra facilities of new table were that it could be raised up or down, that it had a side tilting provision and included a kidney or gall bladder bridge. It only shows that a lot of good surgery can be performed with simple and basic facilities.

Our workshop owner had even made a pair of adjustable knee rests for extended lithotomy position, which let you adjust things like knee position and hip flexion. It was useful during an abdomino-perineal resection of rectum. I soon realised that these local artisans may not have a big qualification but had enough wisdom and common sense to repair complicated equipment and articles; a common trait shared with rural surgeons! Some years later, a local workshop man, Raju, illiterate, self- trained to repair agricultural pump-sets and motors, would regularly 'service' our hydraulic operation table without any service guide book. If it were not for him, the service engineer would have had to come from Bombay. Our overhead OT light could not be positioned easily for a long time. The lamp was supplied from Pune! But this local man dismantled it and repaired it without any difficulty and it worked as though it was new!

Patients came in *tongas* (horse cart), until autorickshaws appeared. Much later ambulances were seen; these were mini vans in which the rear seats were replaced with a stretcher bed. Most of the patients came from surrounding areas by buses. House visits were very uncommon. Even General Practitioners avoided house visits, which I think is a pity. However, I myself might have seen only few patients in their homes.

I had brought most of the instruments for starting general surgery. We bought some more from a representative of a dealer from Bombay. There was no-one to check their instruments if they are as per the standards or had any faults. I bought uterine cervix dilators. Two dilators No. 8 and No.9 were of same thickness but with different numbers! I showed this to the salesman. He thought the problem was with the numbers; not the gauge. "OK doctor, no problem. which number do you want me to change, I will get it done!" without batting an eye as they say. Now I needed funds for recurring expenses like, salaries, electricity, drugs etc. I had only a personal cash reserve of ₹5,000 from the UK earnings when we opened our nursing home (in India, a nursing home typically means a small hospital). My brother chipped in some more. And we started off our practice.

Within a year, a lady needed resection of rectum for cancer and was too poor to go to distant cancer centres. I was confident of performing the surgery, but every other aspect of it was difficult.

Anaesthesia was given by the Government Hospital doctor with ether, with 'Rao's draw over apparatus'. We used the special knee rests that our workshop man had assembled, and I performed both abdominal and perineal parts in a prolonged procedure. For the blood, I had to run to the Government Hospital with the patient's son (donor) to bring fresh blood. She recovered and lived for another 20 years or so and died of some other cause!

Gradually, the practice picked up. In the later years, my brother bought me a good German microscope, a Storz stiff bronchoscope, and also gave me a car to move around. My younger brother who was in the UK bought me a Storz laparoscope, a few anaesthetic accessories, the Epstein-Macintosh-Oxford (EMO) vaporiser, and more. We used the EMO vaporiser for all our surgeries for the next 10-15 years. Our practice, surgical as well as obstetrics thrived and our lease period was nearing its end; we started planning for a purpose-built nursing home.

Soon more practitioners started arriving in Shimoga, bringing in advancements and other specialities, along with some unhealthy practices too. Advances in medicine were of course welcome. They took away some of our patients from those specialities; like orthopaedics and urology. Many years later, the arrival of CT scan, large laboratories, MRI scan and corporate hospitals with very good specialists and super or sub specialists made Shimoga a healthcare centre. However, the greed of the practitioners also brought in practices like tipping *tonga-walas* and auto-rickshaw drivers for diverting patients to their own nursing homes, bribing ambulance drivers to bring all trauma patients to a particular emergency centre, dichotomy (fee-splitting) under the euphemism of referral fees, kickbacks from the laboratories, and such practices, which have all lowered the dignity of the profession. We did not participate in it though that affected our practice to some extent. We also noticed that one could make a decent comfortable living keeping away from all such malpractices.

It is nice to see that despite all the temptation, even now, there still exists a small section of practitioners who value ethical practice above dirty money.

7. The Economics of Private Practice

Someone said that doctors are very bad in money matters. A doctor is happy if he has enough cash in his pocket at the end of the day. He may not realise that his efforts should have brought him more money or that he has spent from his pockets to treat a patient. It was the same with us too. We did not know how to decide consultation fee, bed charges, operation fees, or other service charges. The concept of consultation fee was alien to the Shimoga people of that time; they were used to going to a doctor with a bottle and paying for the 'mixture' given. Nobody was happy to pay ₹3 or ₹5 as a consultation fee, without getting some mixture, pills or injection for it! We had fixed some arbitrary fees for our services. As for us, we were happy as long as the income was more than our expenses. We were very happy on the day when our earnings were Rs.100!

I wanted to know the realistic fees for our nursing home. I requested an accountant friend of mine to guide us in the matter. He called for information on our practice, the number of consultations per month, number of staff and their salaries, number of admissions and the duration of their stay, number of deliveries a month, number of surgeries per month, duration of an operation, cost of the material used per surgery, occupancy rate of the nursing home, and a lot more such information. Though the data supplied by us was not very accurate (my colleagues hesitated to reveal true information about their practice and fee structure), he came up with some revelations.

All of us in Shimoga, then, were charging far below what we should. Our bed charge per day was ₹3; as per his calculation it ought to be a minimum of ₹10 per day without profit. In other words, we were spending ₹7 from our personal earnings, per patient per day on bed costs! The same thing was shown in OT charges, delivery room charges, and so on. He also showed that consultation fee must be a minimum of ₹10 per consultation while we were collecting ₹5. The important message in his calculation was that the bed charges, delivery room, OT charges and service charges must cover the total establishment expenses. Our professional fees (consultation fee, operation fee, delivery charges etc.) must remain separate as our own personal earnings.

In November 1976, the Karnataka State Government brought an ordinance to regulate the nursing home practices. It decided the upper limits of charges by any nursing home. This confused us. Our new charges were far below the ordinance figures; did it mean we may increase ours to that level.

I had formed a Private Consultants and Nursing Home Owners Club (PCNHOC)in Shimoga to encourage co-operation amongst the nursing home owners and to improve relations. I requested all the members to introduce the new fees pattern. The nursing home owners were grateful to the accountant for his nice guidance and were happy to see that our savings increased each month. This experience made me work out the costing of every new activity I planned in the future, though not every gadget or investment would generate income.

It was awkward to collect payment in advance or demand a deposit. Everyone paid the bill at the time of going home and I am happy to say that almost 90 percent of the people cleared their bills honestly. Very few of them asked for a reduction in the bill, and in that case, we did satisfy their demands to the extent possible. Occasionally, the entire bill has been waived off too.

Like most rural surgeons, I learnt ways to reduce the cost of surgery. I practiced knotting of sutures with instruments, like needle holder or artery forceps. This saves a lot on the costly sutures used-cost of special sutures like vicryl was collected from patients. For example, only one 100cm vicryl suture was enough for me to close the lower segment wound of a C-section in two layers and then use the remaining length to close the transverse lower abdominal wound while many others use three of those sutures for the same. I learnt from Mr. Sanford Ryhope (UK) surgeon to use plain sewing cotton thread instead of the costly surgical linen thread. Thread was used for all intra-abdominal ligatures, for bleeders, for serous coat layer of intestinal anastomosis, for skin closure, and such. Later on Dr. Holoch from DTH Germany brought some reusable skin clips that saved me from suturing skin incision and saved some time too. Skin clips available in India need special applicator, are disposable, need special forceps to remove them and are very, very costly. The German clips were of stainless steel, applied by surgeon's hand, left no mark, can be washed, sterilised and reused. I used my set of clips till we stopped our surgeries. I did not pass on the cost of the clips to the patient as they were being used again and again. I never used costly commercial wound closure dressings either; I placed a dry surgical gauze dressing to protect the clips on the wound and fixed it with strips of adhesive plaster. Plastic surgeon Dr Wallace (known for his 'rule of nine' in burns area estimation), said that a minute quantity of serum that exudes from the wound edges dries soon and forms an impervious membrane protecting the wound. So many wounds do not need dressings at all. The Ryhope surgeon Mr. Sanford did not use any dressing at all; I too stopped covering the sutured wound and without any complication. We used the same intravenous infusion (IV) set for more than one day for a single patient! One cardiac surgeon from Mumbai (Dr Ratna Magotra) told us that in their Municipal Hospital, they too recycled the used extra-corporeal transfusion set on a second or even a third patient after due cleaning and sterilisation! I used broad-arm-sling made out of a piece of cloth, instead of proprietary costly arm sling. All this saved a lot of money to the patient who, after all, pays for everything that is used or wasted.

Endoscopy (esophago-gastro-duodenoscopy) was suddenly becoming popular. Over two decades earlier, around 1964, I had seen an earlier endoscope in Ryhope, UK. It was twice the thickness of the current endoscope, as thick as my thumb. The surgeon used it primarily to diagnose, and if needed to take a biopsy of mostly oesophageal strictures and malignancies, stomach and duodenal ulcers and malignancies. The procedure was simple and far superior to the usual barium meal examination that was resorted to till then. No wonder it replaced the barium examination totally. This Ryhope surgeon Mr Sanford had prophetically said at the time that in the future peptic ulcers would be managed by physicians with drugs, and that the surgeons' role would slowly disappear! Those were the days when we and many surgeons in the UK regularly performed numerous gastric surgeries to treat peptic ulcers. That prediction turned out to be true! The Acid-Peptic disorder became a medically manageable disease.

Coming back to endoscopy, the procedure was fairly simple and there were experts conducting short training courses on it. I sat down to work out the cost-efficiency of the investment on the basis of what I had learnt earlier. At that time, the cost of the scope was just over a lakh (₹1,00,000). Add other accessories to it, and the total investment needed would be about a lakh and a half. For some unknown reason, the other practitioners and consultants hesitated referring their patients to a surgeon performing any investigation like endoscopies! That meant I had to depend upon my own referrals for the endoscopy to start generating any income. Number of acid-peptic-disorder patients coming to me were not many, and only some amongst them may need endoscopy; so few that their fees may not be enough to pay off the interest on the investment, leave alone the cost, the depreciation, annual maintenance cost, insurance if any, and so on. Either I had to resort to giving commission for referrals, do unindicated endoscopies, or drop the idea altogether. I chose the latter. Some optimists advised that the number of endoscopies might increase in the future, and then I would start earning from it! But by then the instrument may have to be replaced by a newer version, which could be costlier than the original one. I had learnt this lesson when I bought a small X-ray unit from a physician to help him when he closed his practice. No doubt it was useful, but investment wise, a total liability; I had only my own patients for X-ray and that too, only if it was truly needed, which reduced its use further! Loss due to unused films getting 'fogged' and chemicals becoming wasted was alarming.

I faced a similar situation with laparoscopic surgeries. I was impressed by lap-tubectomy when I attended a local tubectomy camp; NGOs were doing hundreds and thousands of tubectomies in camps. The surgery was done under local anaesthesia through a small hole in the abdomen, was of short duration and the patient could go home the next day. I was confident that I could master it. After my brother brought me a Storz laparoscope, I started performing abdominal lap-tubectomies quite comfortably, as I was quite conversant with monocular vision and work with cystoscopies.. The pneumo-peritoneum in the camps was with fish-tank aerators. So, I too used it and found it acceptable! For some unknown reason, I was not invited for the government tubectomy camps though I had my own laparoscope set, neither did I receive any remuneration for the tubectomies performed by me in the earlier camps! Again, we had to depend upon our own patients only for laparoscopic tubectomies probably because we never paid commissions for any referrals. So, its use was very limited; and if put in terms of cost-effectiveness, it was a real losing proposition! At about the same time, lap-cholecystectomy was getting popular. But the investment needed for the instruments and accessories was quite high. I hardly got a case or two with gall bladder symptoms in a year, and hence did not feel encouraged to invest a huge sum on a lap-surgery setup. At the time my decision appeared to be wise, but then lap surgery progressed to lap-hernia repairs and more. I am not sure if present surgeons can tell whether their investment is paying off or not. There is also the problem of instruments becoming obsolete as newer, better and costlier ones keep coming in. Un-indicated use seems to be a very popular way of earning from the investment on most costly instruments and gadgets.

Some years ago, an enthusiastic anaesthetist friend of mine wanted to introduce a revolutionary idea of a centralized Intensive Care Unit (ICU) to serve the patients from all the nursing homes and practitioners in and around Shimoga. He offered to look after the operated patients from all local nursing homes post-operatively, until the patient is safe to be transferred back to the referring doctor. It was an excellent idea. If all the nursing homes and consultants referred their patients to the central ICU, it was bound to be useful.

A wise friend of the anaesthetist advised him to work out the cost-effectiveness and to also visit a few functioning ICUs in the state. The anaesthetist visited three well-known teaching hospitals that had ICUs. One hospital was planning to close the ICU, as it was perpetually a losing venture; the directors of another private medical college were wondering why at all the college needed an ICU when it was not generating any profits at all. The third medical college was just about making both the ends meet. In other words, ICUs were mainly losing departments. The anaesthetist thanked his friend for opening his eyes and gave up the proposal.

Surprisingly now, every new hospital or nursing home puts a lot of funds into ICUs saying that it is a good income-generating proposal! They invest huge sums of money in buying the equipment and gadgets. However, ICU-trained intensivists and special ICU-trained nurses are hardly seen! ICU guidelines are commonly trespassed. Unscrupulous people find ways and means of generating profits from even losing ventures. An unkind joke that is making the rounds is that: "A vacant bed in an ICU Unit is a strong indication for admission to ICU!".

8. Our Purpose-Built Hospital

Our five-year lease of the *'bhoot bangala'* was about to end. The question arose as to whether to continue in Shimoga or move elsewhere. We had noticed that the rich from Shimoga went to Bangalore for most of their health problems. But the middle-income people, low-income people and villagers were happy with our service. Gradually, some rich too started consulting us. So, we decided to settle in Shimoga with our own nursing home. We could not afford a large site; with the available funds we were happy to settle for a plot of land measuring about 5400 square feet. Now there were bigger problems facing me. We did not have any civil engineer or architect in Shimoga at the time, to plan and build our nursing home. More important was the fact that we did not know the civil (structural) requirements of a nursing home. I could not find this information anywhere (this was obviously before the days of Google). I even visited the local engineering college. They did not know, and directed me to their library. There was only one book, and that too contained scanty, sketchy information on big hospitals, like a district Government hospital. So, I had to be the architect for our proposed nursing home. I had to decide by myself, arbitrarily, the sizes of the wards, OT, delivery room, consultation rooms, waiting area, and so on, based on information gathered from other nursing homes or my own imagination. I had to imagine how much floor area a patient might need, the area for a consultation room, how to design an OT, what other areas may be needed and so on. We had to accommodate all this and more in the site purchased. Then there was the additional equipment to be purchased. If we were to provide all the gadgets recommended, it would have used up almost all the money we had, leaving nothing for the building. So, I had to decide on the bare necessities and hope for future additions as and when feasible. I had a draughtsman – not an architect or engineer, who too had no idea about the requirements of a nursing home. But I had him draw a ground plan on my information and that was the final plan. Nobody knew how to decide how big our septic tank should be (we did not have underground drainage system yet); I had to finally get that information from the Indian Standards Institute in Delhi.

A year or two later the Government brought in a law defining the space requirements for different nursing home activities. Happily, our nursing home satisfied the requirements.

Now the next problem was finance. Providentially for me, the Government had announced a plan to encourage self-employed graduates, by offering 'seed money' of 10 percent of the cost of the whole plan, at low interest rate. Director of the Industrial Training department of the Govt. of Karnataka helped and guided me to draw up a master plan of the new nursing home, that would include future plans too, so that it would increase the total cost of the plan and thus increase the quantum of seed money receivable. I was told that I may build it in two stages; phase I to build what I had planned for the present and then if and when it is found necessary, to continue to phase II, the remaining part. The outlay increased from the originally proposed ₹1.5 lakhs to around ₹5 lakhs. It was accepted, and I received around ₹50,000 as seed money from the Government. This was a low interest rate loan and was to be paid back after clearing the bank loan. We borrowed about ₹1,75,000 from a nationalised bank. We constructed phase I (ground floor only) of the proposed hospital with the bank loan and the seed money.

Lowering Cost of Construction

We tried to cut the costs of construction at every level. A friend of mine put up a brick making unit in his field and used rice husk from his rice mill to burn the brick kilns. A major portion of the wood was *Bharanige,* a hard wood supplied at a very low cost by Shri S. M Pai, an old school classmate of mine in Honnavar. We bought some more from the Government auctions. We got steel windows from Calcutta, and they were cheaper than the locally-made ones. We procured cement directly from the factory, and used red oxide for the flooring, except in the OT where stone flooring was laid. Since we were living in a very small rented house, we built some rooms on the first floor to make our home. That is where I am living even today.

We implemented almost every cost-cutting idea we could think of, and the end-result was that the final cost of our building, around ₹ 2,25,000 which was far less than what was then officially-accepted at the time locally! The Income Tax Officer was suspicious too. He personally inspected the building and was satisfied with the cost-cutting steps taken. The building was ready in eleven months and we moved into it immediately (1976). The new hospital was patient-friendly and comfortable for our work too. It improved our practice and income. I could pay off the bank loan before time, and also pay off the Government loan (seed money) in record time.^b

9. My "Doctor Wife"

I have written earlier that during my job in the medical college, I got married. It was an arranged marriage, maybe because there was no time to fall in love and then get married! Seriously, that was not the reason. I was working far away from her. Usha (nee Usha Shanbhag) was a bright student in her school and she had secured a medical seat on merit in the Mysore Medical College. As the marriage ceremony was being organised, Usha was appearing for her final MBBS examinations in Mysore! Unfortunately, the examinations got postponed for some reason or the other and the results were declared a day before the wedding date. Happily, she had passed. The rural surgeons' survey some years later showed that most of the rural surgeons had doctor wives. Though I had not planned it, it made me happy that my wife too was a doctor. Soon after the wedding I was back at work.

But Usha was yet to complete her internship training. I was working in Davangere medical college; so we managed to get the permission for her to do her internship in the college I was working at. That meant she had to forgo her stipend but we were happy that we could be together and I could help her in her learning process. This was just as well, as I could guide her in some of her work. When she was on casualty duty, there was a small wound to be sutured. Casualty Officers were in the habit of suturing small wounds without local anaesthesia: he told Usha "After all it only needs one or two pricks either way! So do not bother giving local anaesthesia". She was scared and called me. I told her that it is always easy to use the same two pricks to instil local anaesthesia and work comfortably with a cooperating patient; as it often happens, the wound may need a second and sometimes a third stitch! Similarly, it was a common practice to suture an episiotomy wound after vaginal delivery, without local anaesthesia. I asked Usha to use LA. every time When she had to aspirate the chest of pleural fluid, the ward had only a 10ml syringe to be used again and again to aspirate about two litres of the fluid. I had a syringe with a two-way valve specially meant for such 'tapping'. She was happy to use that, drained nearly two litres.

My resignation from the college, and then the decision to start nursing home practice in Shimoga, were far too sudden developments in our lives. I did not know if she had any future plans for post-graduate studies. Starting a nursing home would certainly come in the way of any such plans. My father always felt that obstetrics is a speciality well-suited for women doctors, and that it had great demand in every community and society. He convinced her about it. We started admitting delivery cases. Usha's training in obstetrics was all that she had learnt during the internship period.

The only anaesthetist in Shimoga was a Government Assistant Surgeon 'trained' in anaesthesia, though not qualified. After his duty hours he would visit our nursing home if necessary. Many times, waiting for the Government Anaesthetist was inconvenient; we needed to have our own anaesthetist who would be available at short notice. So, I requested my wife to go and get trained in anaesthesia. She agreed. My cousin Dr. N. M. Prabhu was in the Hubli Medical College. He convinced one of his colleagues, Dr. Deshpande, a Professor of Anaesthesia in Hubli to help us out. Our other request was that she should be well-versed in ether anaesthesia, because, by now my brother working in the UK had brought for me an EMO ether vaporiser. Usha started getting trained and gathering courage and experience. But just at that time we found out that she was pregnant and could not attend to her duties properly. Since anaesthetic gases and the OT atmosphere would not be good for her and the baby's health, she cut short her training and returned home. After delivery, after a short period of 'rest' she joined me in my practice as an anaesthetist for simple and short cases. Later on, we found a qualified anaesthetist, in Dr Rajani Pai, trained in K.E.M.Hospital, Mumbai and Usha was relieved.

Usha was 'self- learning' obstetric practice now and was getting good at it. Occasional problems were solved by a qualified colleague or the old experienced obstetrician, my father. Usha would personally conduct every delivery herself. That is the least she could do, she said, to her patients who put so much trust in her. Her patience and empathy towards the patients made her a popular obstetrician. Soon well-qualified obstetricians arrived in Shimoga. But Usha's practice went on as usual. Not having a post-graduate qualification, Usha felt she should keep her fees below those of the qualified obstetricians. Usha's practice prospered all the same.

I was the surgical arm of her practice. Curettage of uterus (D&C), C-sections, hysterectomies, difficult episiotomies and other gynaecological surgeries were managed by me. There have been situations where we had to call in qualified obstetricians for help. We avoided complicated deliveries, malignancies and major gynaecological procedures.

In our new nursing home, we had overlooked the current (1970s) practice of nursing the new-borns in a separate 'nursery'; this new Western concept was, supposedly, to provide some rest and peace to the tired mother. If we knew of it earlier, I felt we could have provided a room for the nursery to make our nursing home 'modern'. We had followed our, more popular, ancient method of letting the mothers have their baby with them. Mothers were quite happy with the arrangement. But our practice, at the time appeared to be a retrograde step. "Oh! Have you no nursery room!" some would exclaim. However, only a few years later, western Obstetricians said that the 'ancient' Indian method of co-bedding is better for 'bonding' of the baby with the mother, never mind about the peace and rest to the mother! I was pleased to see our age-old wisdom supersede western logic. Dr Antia, retired Professor of Plastic surgery, J. J. Group of Hospitals, Mumbai, often said that Western science needs to be tempered with ancient Indian wisdom. I found the profound meaning of this statement again, some years earlier, though I was not aware of it then. I was travelling in a bus. A youngster sat beside me. During a casual chat, he said he was a farmer and was studying in a college; his father was illiterate and stubborn as he continued to use the natural fertiliser prepared with cow dung, and refused to use chemical fertilisers that increased the yield manifold! 'Organic farming' had not yet caught on then; and I too was unaware of the benefits of organic farming. Yet, I tried telling him that his father would have some special reason for following the old practice. Now, we know that the illiterate father was wiser than the literate son. Another example is the civilised, comfortable, modern commode in our toilets. Now they are trying to popularise the good old Indian style of squatting. The influence of Western medicine has antagonised us against our own ancient, time tested and still useful Ayurvedic sciences. We have closed our mind to even studying the advantages and potential of different aspects of Ayurveda. I believe that we need to re-kindle the national pride in our bosoms.

Usha could devote enough time to her practice as my parents were with us, and that helped us bring up our children with their love and supervision. Having elders in the house is an invaluable asset for the whole family, more so for the younger generation. They instil the values of life, culture, respect for elders, and much more positivity into the children and the succeeding generation. Our hectic life left very little time for us to play around with the children. Yet, our daughter seems to have been influenced by our profession. She took up medicine and is a Paediatrician now. Our son has always been scared of blood and so, is an engineer!

Later when my surgical practice was adversely affected by a medico-legal case, and many corporate hospitals opened in Shimoga,

Usha's practice was our mainstay. It could have continued for more years if it were not for my age and bad health. She could have continued alone too, but then without a surgical arm, she could not practice. So, we retired together.

10. Anaesthesia in Our Practice

In the present days, surgery and anaesthesia go together; it is difficult to imagine surgery without anaesthesia. In the early days of my practice, I had to send away a lady with a breast lump only because there was no one to give general anaesthesia! Whoever wanted general anaesthesia had to 'manage somehow' and carry on. The District Hospital was (and is) a splendid huge hospital with all the main specialities. A lot of planned and emergency surgeries were being performed daily. But they too did not have any qualified anaesthetist at the time. As pointed out before now, an assistant surgeon, who had been trained for anaesthesia would work for all as an anaesthetist. (It was rumoured that in a neighbouring taluk Government Hospital, a ward boy had been administering anaesthesia regularly for years!) Those of us in private practice would utilise the services of this assistant surgeon whenever he was free. Happily, most of the surgical work could be done under spinal anaesthesia and local (regional) anaesthesia; that is why we could survive.

In the very first year of my practice a doctor's son needed circumcision. But we did not have an anaesthetist in the private sector. Another general practitioner who used to be a government doctor before, and had given ether anaesthesia, agreed to give 'open ether' anaesthesia. The procedure is that first ethyl chloride spray is put on the Schimmel Busch mask covering the mouth and nose of the patient and as the patient settles down or 'goes under', ether replaces the ethyl chloride spray. The depth of anaesthesia is decided by the depth of respiration, muscle relaxation, and such factors. With his help I quickly completed the surgery. Such short anaesthesia can be given by most paramedics or doctors with a bit of training. While working in Eastbourne, UK, there were occasions when the casualty sister had to give ether anaesthesia to a fracture patient and I had to 'reduce and set' the fracture!

I started using Local anaesthesia for many procedures. In addition to the usual subcutaneous lumps, I have repaired many inguinal hernias, and performed small plastic procedures for correction. Later I could even do decompression of median nerve at the wrists. One desperate poor girl about ten years old or so, had a wide cleft of upper lip. She and her grandmother refused to go to any distant hospital because of her poverty. I repaired the defect under local anaesthesia. Once the son of our fruit vendor came with a torsion of testis. Instead of waiting for his stomach to be empty for his anaesthesia, I operated on him under local anaesthesia immediately and could undo the torsion within three hours of torsion. I believe the testis was saved, for he became a father later!

I am surprised at the 'rule', if at all there is one, that the operating surgeon himself may not give local anaesthesia; he is required to engage a qualified anaesthetist for the purpose. One Professor of Anaesthesia was emphatic about it. Another Professor of Surgery from Mangalore told me that he always had an anaesthetist stand by whenever he performed surgery under local anaesthesia, however minor it may be! This ignores the fact that thousands and lakhs of dentists disobey this law. A lot of local anaesthesia in emergency rooms, in minor OTs are given by the operating surgeons themselves. The potential of local anaesthesia is being forgotten. Even surgeries like C-section delivery are being comfortably performed with local anaesthesia. One obstetrician from Udupi Government Hospital, Dr. Savitri Daitotha, presented a paper in our ARSI conference, on having performed over 1000 C-Sections with local anaesthesia given by herself. In her initial days of service, finding an anaesthetist was difficult and her senior had taught her the technique of using local anaesthesia. She had become so adept in it that she continued to use it even when there was an anaesthetist available! That is a proven example of an operating surgeon giving anaesthesia himself/herself, which some anaesthesia professors say is medico-legally wrong. One wonders whether the doctor is wrong or the law. But that is a common practice with many rural surgeons due to non-availability of qualified anaesthetists. Even now, there is supposed to be a severe shortage of anaesthetists in our country; about 14,000 anaesthetists for over 31,000 surgeons. In addition, other specialities too need their services. It is alleged that even now, according to the WHO, 60 percent of rural hospitals do not have general anaesthesia facility! Sir Martin Luther King Junior said, "One has not only a legal, but a moral responsibility to obey just laws. Conversely, one has a moral responsibility to disobey unjust laws." I subscribe to that belief.

Lower abdominal surgeries were more in our practice; appendicectomies, hernia repair, haemorrhoids, fissure/fistulae, gynaecological procedures, caesarean deliveries, and such. These were eminently suited to be performed under spinal anaesthesia (sub-arachnoid block). In the initial days, I used to perform the lumbar puncture myself to give this anaesthesia and request my wife to look after the vital parameters of the patient. Soon we became quite adept in it. I continued to do it for many years even when there was a qualified anaesthetist in attendance.

My ability to perform lumbar puncture successfully was put to test when my wife was in labour the first time. This was again, in the very early days of our practice (1971). We had a good obstetrician to attend to the delivery. However, as the baby was 'big' and the membranes had leaked, she felt C-section delivery was immediately needed. As said earlier, there was no qualified anaesthetist in Shimoga. I had no time to organise one from the neighbouring medical college 100 km away. The Obstetrician herself was used to give spinal anaesthesia to her patients in the Government Hospital and then perform surgery. So, we felt she would do the same for us too. Unfortunately, as everything was laid out for the surgery, and my wife, the patient, was lying on the operation table, the obstetrician could not find the right space to inject the lignocaine! We were desperate. Though there were about six more doctors in the OT (Usha's classmates and friends) I was the only other one who had the know-how of the technique of giving spinal anaesthesia. There were no alternatives for me. The only thing for me to do was to try it myself, as two lives were at risk. Fortunately, my attempt succeeded and soon our son was delivered.

The troubles were not over yet. In those early days everyone injected 2 ml of lignocaine for this anaesthesia. I too had injected 2 ml, and Usha is short (height-wise). After the surgery was over, she started complaining of difficulty in breathing, and that, "both her legs were cut and were seen in the corner of the OT," (phantom limb phenomenon). No amount of convincing pacified her. We gave her oxygen by mask and talked to her continuously to convince her that her legs were intact and everything was in order. As the anaesthetic effect wore out, she too settled down and everyone was happy.

In the UK hospital where I worked, there was an anaesthetist, who was an academician to some extent. He taught me the technique of inserting an endotracheal tube, and showed me how the simple open ether anaesthesia is safe, and could be given with an 'ether vaporiser' or the Boyle's apparatus. He had even put together a simple mechanical ventilator (which he called the 'Venntilator' as his name was Dr Venn), in which he had used a small motor to drive the bellows, and ordinary weights from a grocer's store to adjust the pressure of inhaled air mixture! "That," he said, "is a Venntilator for your Jungle Surgery." He took that ventilator to another cardio-thoracic hospital, and took me there too, to show that even open chest surgeries and cardiac procedures are safe with ether vaporiser and his Venntilator! That is how I ventured into doing surgeries with ether anaesthesia given with an ordinary ether vaporiser and later with the EMO vaporiser!

Safety of ether anaesthesia prompted me to even perform abdomino-perineal resection of rectum surgery on a lady. In the initial days of general anaesthesia with ether, the induction would be with ethyl chloride sprayed on a Schimmel Busch mask covering the mouth and nose. The patient had to be restrained until he 'went under' and once the patient was 'under', the endotracheal tube would be inserted and connected to the ether vaporiser. The ether vaporiser was a simple jam bottle named 'Rao's Vaporiser' which also had mechanical bellows for respiratory support. Oxygen was derived from the air in the mixture. We had a lot of problems with the supply of medical oxygen. It could take up to a month just to get one empty cylinder refilled by the British Oxygen company from Bangalore (275 km from Shimoga)! That too, with a lot of red tape! So, most of the times we had to use air ether mixture for general anaesthesia. A colleague of mine even found out that, as per WHO, industrial oxygen is good enough for human consumption in an emergency.

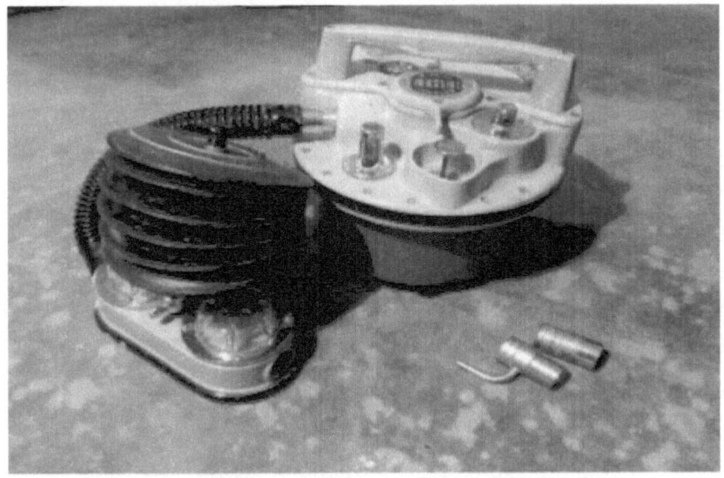

Figure 1: Epstein, Macintosh, Oxford vaporiser (EMO)

Surgeries took a longer time with ether anaesthesia and at the end everyone in the OT would smell strongly of the ether. When we returned home, our children would run away from us because of the ether smell! I have done most of the abdominal surgeries with such general anaesthesia. A good anaesthetist would even use muscle relaxants just like in any other type of anaesthesia.

Many times, waiting for the Government Hospital Anaesthetist would be inconvenient. So, as pointed out earlier, Usha had trained herself for anaesthesia and helped me in emergencies until we had a qualified anaesthetist. Dr Rajani Pai was the first properly-qualified, private anaesthetist in Shimoga. She had trained in G. S. Medical College and K. E. M. Hospital, Bombay. She had married a doctor in Shimoga, and started practicing here. She could work with EMO too. Suddenly, all our anaesthesia problems were solved. Usha, my wife, was the anaesthetist for small surgeries, and the new anaesthetist was there for the rest.

We did all sorts of surgeries with the EMO outfit, abdominal, neck, orthopaedic, Ob&Gy, paediatric and so on. With a good anaesthetist, it was as good as a Boyle's unit. I am not convinced about the fire and explosion hazard with ether in the OT. However, we were careful as long as we used the EMO. When I wanted to install a window air-conditioner (A/C) unit, the VOLTAS refused to sell one to us saying that the induction motor spark of the unit is a fire hazard in an atmosphere of inflammable anaesthetic gases that are used during surgery. By that observation, ordinary electric switches also are to be banned as also the fans and suction units! Most the OTs that I visited after those days had window A/C units, sparking switches, some even had fans and ordinary electric wall switches. So, we too installed an A/C unit in our OT. We have not regretted it.

Later on, we had a halothane vaporiser for the EMO too. We used the EMO for the next 15-20 years. By then, many more anaesthetists started coming into the private sector in Shimoga; but they were not familiar with the EMO. For some reason, medical college anaesthesia professors looked down upon the EMO outfit. That is when we purchased a Boyle's machine. Besides Dr Rajani Pai too was busy assisting her doctor husband. So, the EMO gradually went out of use. Now our Boyle's unit too is outdated! Recently I donated them both to the Anaesthesia department of the Shimoga Institute of Medical Science (SIMS) as a museum pieces.

11. Erratic Power Supply and Training Our Own Nurses

Power supply in our town was very erratic. Though the Electricity Board was expected to inform the users before switching off power, they hardly did that. For us, that was a big unpredictable set back, especially for planning surgery. One evening, we had to perform a C-section delivery. All was well until incision was made on the uterus to deliver the baby. The lights went off suddenly. Pitch dark in the OT. I had to deliver the baby's head but could not see it. Someone switched on a torch and somehow, I extracted the baby. But we needed the suction apparatus to suck out the blood and liquor. Blood and liquor started flooding the abdominal wound making a mess of the surgical drapes and OT floor. We used a mechanical foot-suction-pump but that was not enough either. The torch light was not adequate to proceed with the surgery. Green-Armytage forceps controlled the bleeding from the lower segment incision. I was desperate, though the emergency was under control. Work was difficult without light in the OT. We continued under the torchlight. We used abdominal mops to empty the blood and liquor. Someone ran to bring a petromax lamp (one that works on kerosene pumped under pressure to light an incandescent filament). By the time it arrived, the messy surgery was almost over. The placenta was removed. The residual blood and liquor in the abdominal cavity were mopped up with abdominal mops. Then the abdomen was closed.

Now, like the dramatic arrival of the police after the shoot-out in movies, power arrived for us!

When we moved in to the new hospital, it was a totally new, enjoyable feeling of nursing home practice. We wanted to install an electric power generator (dynamo) as power cuts were frequent. I purchased a small, imported Honda generator, that even a nurse may be able to start. But corrupt officials continued to create unnecessary problems; the Electricity Board raised many objections including a demand for a lab certificate from the manufacturers (from Japan) before they can permit its use! Anyone may guess the reason behind all this. They even found faults with the earthing provided. Luckily for us, a sensible electrical inspector was there who realised that the unreasonable demands were unfair and that the earthing was far better (he tested it with a meter) than that in most other buildings. He was good enough to give us permission for the generator use. Over the years, we installed an uninterrupted power supply (UPS) unit and batteries, which was even more useful.

Next was the problem of nurses and other technical staff. No one was readily available. Those who pass from a government nursing school have to compulsorily take up jobs in government hospitals only. Those that passed out of the few private nursing schools elsewhere had their sights on faraway places like the USA or Middle East. So, most of us private practitioners trained our own nurses. They were 'trained' nurses, not 'qualified' or 'registered' nurses. We hired some local girls – one was a school drop-out too – and trained them to our needs. This implied that we taught them 'nursing' as we knew it. Later still, the Government insisted on qualified nurses in private establishments. It was unfair to sack those working with us. Even now, it was difficult to find qualified nurses. The private practitioners conducted proficiency examinations for the current nurses in employment and those who passed were given 'certificates of training'. The authorities were requested to accept these nurses as trained ones. I believed that our nurses were as good as any qualified ones, and some of them were even better in their work and duties. My OT assistant, who also looked after the sterilisation of instruments and preparing the OT for surgery, was a high-school dropout. He passed SSLC exam while working with us. In those days we could not find trained or certified OT technicians. We had to train one for ourselves, just as we did for our nursing staff. This boy picked up the work so well that he was my first assistant for most surgeries till I retired. He handled instruments too with such expertise that he always had them ready in his hand even before I asked for them. His efficiency in sterilizing operation instruments and other material could be seen when I performed a series of surgeries without antibiotics.

The Government had insisted on minimum wages for all the staff. I was in favour of instituting the minimum wages; after all, satisfied staff is an asset to the establishment. But many in the PCNHOC did not agree. In Shimoga, ours was one of the very few nursing homes that paid the minimum wages as per the law. The number of employees on our pay roll was smaller than that needed for obligatory Employees' Provident Fund (EPF) contributions, yet we had voluntarily started that too. I had also started the Gratuity Fund, so I believe that our staff was happy working for us. They all had some pension too.

12. Practice Without Laboratory, Radiology and Blood Bank. Autologous Blood Transfusion

One other difficulty we had to put up with was the lack of investigative facilities. When I chose Shimoga for our practice, I did not realise that a district headquarters, having the best district hospital in the state, would be without a clinical laboratory, blood bank or proper radiology service. So, we had to start our own small clinical lab with Sahli's haemoglobinometer, a microscope, hand centrifuge for urine examination, a spirit lamp, test tubes, and such. We performed our own tests, examined stools, urine, blood cell counts, and more. The satisfaction of finding live amoeba in the stools of a patient suspected to have amoebic colitis, or finding ova of worms, pus cells in urine, examining blood film, and so on, was unique. We could even identify the eggs of thread worms from the perineum of a patient. We were no experts, but we became familiar with some common laboratory tests.

About five years later, a biochemistry technician started a clinical laboratory, but he lacked in bacteriology and histopathology, both of which came to Shimoga some years later. Later still, a local girl, Dr Shanthi MD Pathology, dependable pathologist came to Shimoga and established well-equipped ESSEM laboratory. After that, many more laboratories opened in Shimoga with their own pathologists, and six to seven corporate and large hospitals with their lab and pathologists too!

When we started practice, Shimoga had one radiologist but he was doing mostly plain X-rays, some barium meal studies, the occasional cholecystogram, and rarely intravenous pyelograms (IVP), and that too, only when the patient's doctor went with the patient to inject the medium! Generally, the commonest X-rays were of the chest, bones and joints, and abdomen.

If I had reduced and set a bone fracture, it would be immobilised in a POP cast. Then, the patient would be sent to the radiologist to take X-ray pictures to 'check' if the positioning of the fragments was acceptable. If it was not, the plaster had to be cut open and re-reduction was tried once again. It was a time when C-arm X-ray unit in the OT was unheard of, and so was CT scan! However, now we have many corporate hospitals and some multi-speciality group hospitals each having its own C-arms, CT unit and MRI units too. I for one am quite illiterate with CT scans and MRI pictures, and did not feel their absence then. But now, CT scan has overtaken clinical examination of the patient. One instance that amused me a lot was when a surgeon asked for a radiogram of the abdomen instead of a rectal digital examination, to see if the patient was constipated! I too had a small X-ray unit for some time. I found out that the number of patients genuinely needing an X-ray was so low that our films got fogged in storage and chemicals became out-of-date (or ineffective after long periods). Now, progress of a patient is decided with daily CT scans! The cash till has pushed clinical medicine out.

It is difficult to imagine surgical practice, especially emergencies, without the backup of a blood bank. When I started practice in Shimoga, there was no blood bank. All those patients who were likely to need blood for their surgeries had to go elsewhere! What about the emergencies? We tried our best to save patients with blood volume expander fluids like Haemaccel and normal saline, and sometimes with blood donated by a relative and cross-matched by the doctor!

However, the Government Hospital had a 'blood bank', which was not a bank in its true sense because there were no stocks of blood at any time. A sister collected the blood of a donor, found out his blood group, checked if it 'matched' (was compatible) with the patient's blood and if yes, she collected the blood of the donor for transfusion. The method is now called Unbanked Direct Blood Transfusion (UDBT). This 'bank' was under the command of the District Surgeon (DS). During an emergency situation in my hospital, the DS refused to permit the relatives of our patient to donate blood there! For some unknown reason, he had decided that private surgeons would not be permitted to use this facility. Now government hospitals look to private blood banks for blood units. Of course, we continued to use the 'old bank' by cajoling the blood bank sister and getting her help for our patients. But in emergencies, it could be difficult indeed. Now, we have more than two private blood banks and their services are quite satisfactory. They even supply blood to the Government Hospital patients. Even blood components are now available when needed.

I had heard and read about 'autologous blood transfusion' that is collecting patient's blood and preserving it to be used during the surgery on the same patient. The ABT has been successfully used in many cases of ruptured tubal gestations. I found that it was a doable process. So, I researched and put together a set of things that were needed for the procedure, and kept them sterile and ready in our OT – a large stainless steel tea strainer, a funnel (glass or steel) into which the strainer would fit, small pots to scoop blood from the abdomen, a larger pot or pan to collect the strained blood, sets of surgical gauze in four layers and anticoagulant citrate dextrose (ACD) bottles for blood collection. Those were the days when the blood was collected in glass bottles with anticoagulants. I always had two bottles in our OT. It was not long before I had to resort to that method.

A general practitioner came to me one morning with his niece, who was to go to Bangalore that morning, but suddenly developed abdominal pain. She said she fainted too. Yes, she had missed her periods also. I suspected ruptured ectopic gestation; physical examination confirmed the diagnosis. But this was before the days of urine test for pregnancy and ultrasonography. To be sure of the need to do an emergency surgery, I decided to do an abdominal (peritoneal) tap. Frank blood filled the syringe! Immediate surgery was decided. But what about the blood? I urged the doctor to try for blood from the Government Hospital bank, and in the meantime, I would try to salvage as much blood as possible from patient's abdomen to re-transfuse it in her circulation.

As soon as the abdomen was opened, dark blood and clots started flowing out. This was not contaminated blood. I started scooping out the blood and pouring it onto the four-layered gauze in the funnel. The filtered blood was collected in the larger pot. If we left the blood in the pot for long, it would clot, and so we frequently transferred it to the blood collection bottles. This bottle had to be lightly agitated all the time so that the anticoagulant mixed with the blood thoroughly. Each ACD bottle had 150 ml anti-coagulant, and could take 300 ml blood, making a total volume of 450 ml. Now this bottle was ready for re-transfusion into the patient immediately! In this patient, I could salvage three bottles of blood that could be transfused back into her immediately. Another bottle and a half of clots had to be discarded.

I have used this method in 15 patients, and have salvaged more than three units each from six of them, all with ruptured ectopic gestations. All that good blood would otherwise have been thrown away. No one had any complications or side reactions. This method is very useful when blood is not available immediately. In fact no blood bank can supply blood quicker than the ABT supplied the first unit collected from the abdomen. The advantages are many: the salvaged blood does not need time-consuming tests, is available immediately, and costs just as much as the cost of ACD bottles. However, one must ensure that contaminated blood from the source is not salvaged.

Now, blood bank rules have made this method illegal!

13. OT in a Rural Hospital; and Surgery Without Antibiotics

In those times, there was no formalised information, such as standards and protocols, on how a small surgical Operation Theatre should be – the size, equipment, organisation, supplies like linen, requirements like sterilisation, and so on. Without these, it was difficult for rural surgeons and owners of small hospitals to setup an OT, and also to verify whether an OT satisfied the requirements or not.

A book on advances in surgery, around 1965, discussed the civil plan of an OT (the actual room) only. Just like different medical colleges and doctors differed on the sterilisation process for instruments, so too did information on preparing an OT for surgery. We all knew that an OT has to be 'clean', 'comfortably roomy' and 'aseptic'; but the definition of each of these words varied from person to person. Yet surgeons continued to perform surgeries in their OTs not knowing the exact cause of infections when they occurred. Nobody seemed to know the relation between the types of surgical procedures and the size and quality of the OT preparation. People suggested we invest on costly things like the latest air filters, UV light, airflow fixtures and planum ventilators just to be on the safer side.

Some of us might have heard of famous 'Indian, Hindu rhinoplasty' story. The story goes that a certain Cowasjee, who was a bullock cart driver for the British army in India, was caught by the army of king Tippu Sultan of Mysore, a sworn enemy of the British. Cowasjee was punished by cutting his nose off. When he returned home, Cowasjee went to a brick maker near Pune, who created a skin flap from the forehead down – and with that a brand new nose for Cowasjee! This allegedly happened in 1793. This procedure had been practiced over thousands of years from the time of Sushruta (about 600 BC) who had introduced the technique of rhinoplasty. What impressed me, more than the reconstruction of the nose, was the fact that the surgery was performed by a brick maker, not a medical man. He might not even have known of concepts like sterilisation of equipment, asepsis as we know now, and yet even more importantly, the wound healed without any antibiotics. The procedure itself would have been performed in the open, no doubt with bare hands and mostly without current aseptic measures! There surely is a message here to us all. The world of western medicine might not recognise Ayurveda as a proper medical science; yet it cannot deny many of its achievements. For instance, how could they avoid or control infections in surgical wounds? They used to perform cataract surgery, abdominal surgery, piles, fistula surgery, and much more. It potentially means that a man's body has enough strength to fight off any infection of the operation wounds! Then, why can't more of us use the same power of the human body to ward off infections in simple and clean surgeries now? I believe that if we try, we can. It would save the money spent on antibiotics!

Our OT was an ordinary room, 14 x 16 ft., with two windows, both open to the outside. We used to 'prepare' the OT before each surgery. That involved a thorough cleaning of the room, mopping the floors walls and furniture with phenyl. Since the OT air might be contaminated by organisms from the OT staff, surgeons or patients themselves, we would open the windows to let out the OT air and to let in fresh air from outside. The density of bacterial population in outside air was likely to be far below than that in our OT and the bacteria themselves would be less pathogenic compared to the bacteria from hospital staff, patients' infected wounds, hospital air etc. Besides, a study has shown that there is no correlation between air contamination and the occurrence of surgical site infection (SSI). Though wound contamination does occur in 10-40 percent of the surgical procedures, fortunately they rarely lead to SSI[1]. However, if and when a procedure involved an infected wound, our OT would be fumigated with formalin, all the OT furniture and fixtures would be cleaned with phenyl once again, and so on.

Initially, some of us wore OT dress, but 'circulating' nurses – those that ran around during an operation – did not, as they also had to attend to ward calls. (Such multitasking was essential to reduce the number of nurses and, in turn, the establishment expenses). Some years later, I had a split A/C for our comfort, which only recycled the OT air, but did not have planum ventilation, OT air exchanges under pressure, UV light to sterilise the air, and such things. The surgical metal instruments, gowns and linen were meticulously autoclaved. We used the 3M (Bowie Dick) autoclave tape to check the sterility of the load in the autoclave. On the rare occasion of performing a laparoscopic tubectomy, we sterilised the disassembled laparoscope in a formalin chamber.

In short, from academic points of view, our OT and our practices had many shortcomings for any type of surgery! But adequacy of asepsis by these simple methods was amply demonstrated to us by Dr Ratna Magotra, a cardio-thoracic surgeon from K.E.M. Hospital, who performed an open-heart surgery in the Udhampur District Hospital, Jammu, during the annual conference of ARSI. That hospital, like most district hospitals, did not have any

---

[1] Birgand G, Azevedo C, Toupet G, *et al* Attitudes, risk of infection and behaviours in the operating room (the ARIBO Project): a prospective, cross-sectional study *BMJ*
Open 2014;**4**:e004274. doi: 10.1136/bmjopen-2013-004274

of the sophisticated OT sterilisation measures. Similarly, a spine surgeon told me how he performed a spine correction surgery in a small private hospital in a tribal area of Gadchiroli, Maharashtra. There too they did not have sophisticated gadgets for OT air sterilisation.   So, our methods were not wrong, obsolete or unscientific after all. *WHO Guidelines for Safe Surgery* (2009) supports our views even further.

In the UK, I had worked with surgeons who practiced what they believed in, even though it might not be in the text books. I have written earlier about how a surgeon, Dr Sanford never used skin paint before taking an incision. I was taken aback when I was asked in the final FRCS examination about exactly the same topic – using skin paint before surgery. I boldly told the examiner about the practice we practiced in the UK hospital I worked at, and the examiner was gracious enough to accept it! I admired his humility. I felt that I too should talk about our OT in Shimoga, and show, how safe surgery could be performed in it despite the shortcomings.

During an Association of Surgeons of India (ASI) conference, around 1995, I happened to say that air in an OT was not a cause for surgical site infection as many surgical camps were held in school classrooms used as make shift OTs, and incidence of infection in these camps was not high. Secondly, most of us conducted operations in ordinary rooms in rented houses that were used as nursing homes, and yet our infection rates were low. My statements enraged a senior surgeon who later became the president of the ASI (not that the office reflects the depth of surgical knowledge or maturity of thinking). He shouted that I was misleading the senior students into wrong practices! That enraged me. On returning home, I did a prospective study in my own small nursing home to support my statement.

Prospective Study Of Surgery Without Antibiotics

I made a proper selection of cases for the study. Only healthy individuals were selected for the study. A few healthy persons with potential infection were also selected. I excluded from the study those who were too old, too ill, had associated diseases, or also those hernias that needed mesh-repair.

T he patients were preferably admitted one day prior to the day of planned surgery and all the usual pre-operative procedures were carried out as they were done in our nursing home. After all, the goal was to find out if the procedures we followed in our nursing home were adequate or not. The surgeons' and OT sisters' hands were scrubbed with carbolic soap and water thrice, and when available with antiseptic scrub. But I found simple soap and water scrub was adequate for our purpose. Tincture Iodine was used to paint the operation area and around it. Simple drapes were used to cover areas around the operation site. Skin-wound- edge towels were not used. I tried my best to focus religiously on the Halstead tenets: gentle handling of tissues and organs, sharp anatomic dissection, perfect haemostasis, thorough excision of devitalised tissue, avoidance of dead space and tension, and use of non-irritant sutures. The skin was closed with simple interrupted cotton thread sutures. When infection was suspected, antibiotics were used.

List Of Surgeries Performed For The Study		
1	Hernias	78
2	Acute and chronic appendicitis	56
3	Breast lumps and other tumours	25
4	Thyroidectomy	7
5	Planned C-section deliveries	5
6	Hysterectomies	3
	Total	174

Of the total of 174 cases, 165 healed without the use of antibiotics. Only two patients who had tachycardia even on day-3 post op, received antibiotics and they healed. Another two showed wound infection when suture or clips were removed; they too healed with the use of antibiotics. One patient with muscle-cutting incision had wound infection despite the use of antibiotics from post-op day 1. Interestingly, one boy had a gangrenous (grey) turgid appendix, but it was still intact, that is, it had not ruptured. After it was removed as a whole carefully, without rupturing, he too healed without antibiotics. I believe that 165 successes out of 174 is a good enough proof that our OT was fit for our surgical procedures!

This proves that it is quite possible and feasible to perform clean surgical procedures without antibiotics and without sophisticated gadgets like air filters, in the surgical OT. We underestimate the body's innate ability to fight a small number of bacteria that may inadvertently land into the operation wounds.

Wounds of clean surgeries are essentially clean and capable of healing without antibiotics. They tend to be infected only due to faulty sterilisation of instruments, bad surgical techniques, bad OT discipline, and such factors. There was also a study, which reported lack of evidence to prove that SSI was due to OT air contamination. However, major surgeries – transplants, brain, cardiac and orthopaedic surgeries – need special and better equipped OTs.

14. Some Unusual Experiences: The Power of Prayer

It may sound unscientific to some of you, but I sincerely believe in prayers and *japas* (chants). In the last 80 odd years of my life, I have seen many incidences that could not be explained by 'rational' or evidence-based science. Before every surgery, I used to chant a prayer to Lord Dhanvantari, as I scrubbed my hands. And I believe, regardless of what anyone else may think, that this sincere prayer made even difficult surgeries doable. I have heard a cardiac surgeon confess to a similar experience.

When I was in primary school, our astrologer said that, as per my *kundali* (horoscope), I would be "good with my hands" and that I would use sharp cutting tools. He predicted that I would become either a sword-wielding soldier or, being the son of a doctor, a surgeon! I have great regard for our horoscopic findings and predictions. It all depends upon how good the astrologer is. It is like diagnosing a difficult medical problem. A clever physician may diagnose it correctly whereas others may not. I have written how an FRCP physician in the UK in 1963 analysed and discussed the full case history of a patient just by looking at a chest X-ray; he was not told about any symptoms, history or any other investigations earlier. He discussed the findings in the X-ray and then correctly diagnosed a rare medical condition of the patient! No one else in the room had even thought of that condition!

I could write about many verified horoscopic predictions during my lifetime alone. The latest one was about me, again. I had decided that I would retire at the age of 80, around 2015. But my horoscope prediction in 2015 was that I could not retire until I was 84 years old, that is around 2019. I had actually closed my hospital when I was 80, but the horoscope reader had said that my stars would push me to work against my decision! That was exactly what happened. Though our hospital was closed, my wife continued with her consultations only. Her pregnant patients who required a C-section insisted that I do the surgery! The closure of our hospital upset them. We had to give in to their requests and I performed the surgeries in a nearby hospital. This stopped all of a sudden when I reached 84, in 2019, when my heart problems started, I had to stop everything.

Coming back to my faith in *japa,* let me tell you about a case in which I believe that *japa* contributed a lot, or was responsible for saving a patient from death.

It was in the very second year of our starting our practice (1972). I went to see a 49-year-old man from a very respectable family of this region, at his house, as he was too ill to come to our consultation room. He had had gall stones, diagnosed in Bangalore many years ago and he had received some medical treatment for it. He had to take that awful-tasting and nauseating concoction from pharmacopeia for many days and that experience had made him phobic to allopathic doctors! He now trusted only Ayurvedic medicine. He had had abdominal pain for many days, but had kept away from allopathic medicine. His condition deteriorated fast and he had to agree to being examined by me. He had vomited for some days earlier, and the pain was getting worse. I found him to be cachectic, in an emaciated, unhygienic condition, and his oral hygiene too was very bad. Clinical examination suggested intestinal obstruction, and if that was confirmed by an X-ray picture of the abdomen, immediate surgery was indicated. I discussed the poor prognosis, and if they agreed to surgery, I asked them to bring the patient to our nursing home with the X-ray.

Next day, they came, and the X-ray confirmed the obstruction. They agreed to the surgery too, but requested that it be performed at 12.30 am that night. They were very conservative and religious, and believed in doing all important actions only at the auspicious time according to their horoscopes – and 12.30 am was the auspicious time given to them by their astrologer. Since we did not have any work either, I agreed to their request. There was no way of assessing the patient's electrolytes, or other parameters. I, once again, impressed upon the relatives the very poor prognosis of the procedure because of lack of facilities such as a blood bank, laboratory and also because the patient's health was critically low. After the successful surgery, they told me that they too did not think that the patient would survive the surgery; they had already made all the preparations at the cremation site for a quick cremation of the body taken directly from the nursing home!

Laparotomy was performed under general (ether) anaesthesia. The abdomen was full of thick, oily, slimy, fluid. It was all sucked out. Two tubercular strictures, one in the jejunum and one at the terminal ileum were found. In view of the poor general condition of the patient, a quick new passages were established to bypass the strictures. The abdomen was closed. Antibiotics and anti-tuberculosis treatment were begun.

His recovery was very slow and worrisome to all of us. We played blindly with IV fluids like Hermin and Ringer's Lactate to make up for any possible electrolytic imbalances. His abdomen became soft, he passed some gas from below and we even removed the nasogastric tube. We all felt very optimistic about his recovery.

Suddenly, on 17th day after the surgery, he had a 'sinking feeling'. The next day was no better, and so we called in a physician. He suggested six-hourly Hydrocortisone and Coramin as a desperate last measure. We also told the relatives that, for some reason the patient was not responding to the medicines, and that we were worried about his health. Two days later, the patient became delirious. He was put on oxygen by mask; the concept of intensive care had not arrived in Shimoga then, and monitors were not available too. The patient's relatives were requested to get a unit of blood, if possible, as a last resort.

Once again, the relatives had an unusual request. They had a *guru* coming from Kerala, whom they have a lot of faith in. He wanted to perform *Mahamrutyunjaya Japa* near the bed of the patient. According to the *guru*, the patient was going through an extremely difficult, life-threatening period in his life. This period would worsen and end at 4 pm that day. Anything could happen during that time. So, the *guru* wished to perfor the *Mahamrityunjaya Japa* till the critical 4 pm. If the patient survived that period, he would fully recover, the *guru* assured.

Since we and our science had nothing more to give, I readily agreed to their request. I was in my consultation room, visiting the patient now and then. I could see him sinking slowly. First, he called his son to tell him of their commitments, but soon had no strength to speak. Then, he called his wife and daughter, and only blessed them as he was too weak to speak. The *guru* went on doing his *japa*.

4 pm passed, and nothing bad had happened. The *japa* too ended. Someone had managed to get 'O' group blood, and we started transfusing that. The patient continued to be in the same state. He had survived the critical period. Did the *japa* have any role in his survival? I cannot say. But, two days later the patient felt better and showed improvement. He improved day by day. He recovered fully albeit slowly. He went home almost two months after the surgery, and lived for over 20 years after that. It is difficult to prove that the *japa* saved the patient; however, it is equally difficult to deny its role.

It may sound unscientific to say that I too believe in such 'occult' phenomenons, but when I think that some years later, we had another similar patient with tubercular abdomen who met with a sad ending, I am led to think maybe the *japa* did have some effect.

(Currently, ICMR is funding a project to chant the *Mahamrityunjaya Mantra* to aid brain-injury patients in Ram Manohar Lohia Hospital, Delhi.)

15. Good Deeds Bring Good Returns

"It is one of the most beautiful compensations of life that no man can sincerely try to help another without helping himself."-

Ralph Waldo Emerson

I have often heard that good deeds bring good returns; but I hardly imagined that I would see it proved in an episode of my own life itself.

When I was in the UK, in 1963, my father had a severe heart attack. Because of poor communication facilities of that time I learnt about it some days later through an aerogramme. My mother was alone at home. My elder brother and sister who were far away came and looked after my father until he became fit enough to 'look after himself'. After their departure, my weak father found it difficult to manage his own daily chores; he needed someone to be with him 24x7. We had a neighbour Shri V. P. Kamat, who was very dear to my father and to us too. After the departure of my brother and sister, he offered to tend to my father. He closed his shop and was with my father day and night for many days, until my father could take care of himself all by himself. Never bothering about his losses, Venkateshanna looked after my father – in my mother's words, "like a son," performing all clean and unclean chores. I learnt all this only after my return from the UK. When I met him, he said what he did was the least he could do for their favourite and dear family *'doctormam'*! He dismissed his help as a neighbourly duty, not mentioning a word about his losses or difficulties! I wanted to pay him back for his invaluable, timely and selfless service, but could not decide how.

As I moved to Shimoga and set up my practice, all that was forgotten. Many years passed by. One day my father had a sudden urge to visit Ankola, for no special reason. He felt like meeting some of his old friends. I went with him on this unplanned visit. After meeting another friend, we headed to visit our dear neighbour, Venkateshanna who had once helped my father so selflessly. When we arrived at his house, the household was very tense. "Doctor mam (our way of saying doctor uncle), we have a big problem that we do not know how to solve," our friend said with tears in his eyes.

It is a tradition amongst most families here that the first delivery of their daughter is conducted in her parents' place (or, in other words, the parents have to look after the first delivery of their daughter). Our friend's daughter had come all the way from Bombay to unequipped Ankola for her first delivery. Now, she was in labour for the past three days, and yet there was no sign of the baby coming out. We knew the nurse Meerabai Gaitonde , in attendance; she was a well-known, qualified and registered staff nurse, trained in J. J. Group of Hospitals, Bombay when I was the student there. She said that baby was in the outlet but the mother was too exhausted to push it out. So, they were planning to go to Karwar as there was no obstetrician in Ankola. Unfortunately, there were no ambulances in Ankola either to take the lady in such an advanced stage of labour to the Karwar hospital. They had to hire a taxi. But there were none available immediately. So, the situation was desperate. Survival of the baby was already doubtful, and the mother's life could be in danger too.

When doctors practice alone, they often face situations where they have to take the final decision regarding a patient's treatment despite all the risks it might involve, notwithstanding the limitations of their own knowledge, training, equipment and infrastructure.

"You do not study to pass the test; you study to prepare for the day when you are the only thing between a patient and the grave."

Mark Reid

Here in Ankola, the day of my test had arrived. I seemed to be the only one who had a chance to save the mother and the baby. While occasionally helping my wife with her obstetric cases, I had experience of applying outlet forceps to pull out the baby. I requested the nurse to take me to the patient. The head of the baby was indeed in the outlet. So, outlet forceps extraction was needed. But there was no one in Ankola to do that. I knew the patient from childhood as they were our neighbours. I said I might be able to help, while they waited for the taxi. I talked to the mother to boost her morale. I explained to her the procedure I was going to try and that she need not worry. She agreed to my help. Whatever the nurse had said was true. The foetal heartbeat was good and strong too. I asked the nurse if a pair of outlet forceps were available anywhere in Ankola. Luckily for us, she carried one herself. The forceps was quickly sterilised by boiling. Happily, she also had lignocaine for local anaesthesia and catgut for suturing episiotomy. But she did not have sterile gloves. I prepared myself with thorough cleaning of hands and forearm with soap and water. I had to work without gloves.

Using the available clean-not sterile linen and saris as drapes, I infiltrated the perineum with lignocaine to be able to give a generous episiotomy. The baby's scalp was visible. I gently applied the outlet forceps and gave a gentle pull. The baby came out easily and suddenly with a gush of liquor. The baby cried immediately, much to the relief of all. I waited for the placenta to come out, and made sure that the uterus had contracted well. I do not remember if the nurse gave her Methergine injection. I then sutured the episiotomy with catgut that the nurse supplied. The mother was happy that the baby was safe and that the whole episode was over. The gloom that had enveloped the household disappeared and everybody cheered for the new arrival. Venkteshanna shed tears of joy and relief.

Many 'blunders' in the aseptic procedure were, unavoidably, committed during this delivery. These stories sound like the old English novels where the doctor performs an appendicectomy on a dinner table in the patient's house. Both prove the same point – that desperate situations need desperate measures!

However, I have not yet found a rational answer to the question of why my father decided to go to Ankola on that particular day. It could only be the 'beautiful compensation of life' for the selfless service rendered by our neighbour – the happy twist of destiny.

Here is another unusual situation, where innovation alone saved the day! An old general practitioner, who happened to be my father's classmate, had come to consult me about a small lump in his epigastrium. Obviously, it was a small epigastric hernia. He had consulted a leading surgeon in Hubli and strangely, he was advised to give up rice in his meals as a treatment for it. I was surprised, no doubt, and told him that it could be treated with a small surgical procedure even under local anaesthesia. He agreed and the next day it was duly repaired under local anaesthetic infiltration. During his stay, he told me some of his experiences as an obstetrician; I came to know later that he too was well-known for his skill in delivering babies! Once, when he had gone to the neighbouring town, he was called up for a delivery that was not progressing. He faced the same situation that I had faced; foetal head was seen in the perineum but not coming out. Unfortunately, there were no outlet forceps or gloves either. So, he washed his hands well, grasped the scalp hair of the baby tightly and tugged with all his strength. Slowly, the baby came out alright. But he was surprised to see the placenta too had come out with the baby. He found out that the umbilical cord was hardly four inches in length! Happily, both the mother and the baby were saved!

In rural practice, we are often caught in peculiar situations, not usually found in text books, where, we need to tread on the proverbial untrodden path, and use all the ingenuity we can muster to give relief to the suffering patient.

16. Betel Nut Piece in the Air Passage

In rural practice, unexpected surgical emergencies crop up very frequently. Whether one can manage the problem depends upon the problem and the ingenuity of the rural surgeon. That is why multi-speciality training goes a long way in rural surgical practice. Some problems are so unique that a doctor might face it only once in his or her entire career, yet the satisfaction of being prepared and equipped to manage the situation is priceless! Often the investment on equipment may not even be recovered.

I have mentioned earlier, about a Dr Venn in the UK. Our hospital there used to have many elderly patients. Many of them developed respiratory infections after surgery; the patient was too weak to cough out the secretions, and that creates complications. Dr Venn used to take those patients to the OT and suck out the bronchial secretions to make them breathe easier. He showed me, and then taught me how to introduce a stiff bronchoscope in a conscious patient by just spraying local anaesthetic in the throat. Some patients would still be under the influence of anaesthesia; others wide awake! Bronchoscopy made it easy to suck out the secretions from the bronchial tree making breathing easier. Of course, it did create some discomfort to the patient, but with the patient's cooperation, the procedure could be done successfully. This confidence to be able to pass a stiff bronchoscope under local anaesthetic spray in the throat, emboldened me to buy a bronchoscope for my practice in India without even bothering to do some study regarding the scope for such a procedure or work out the cost-effectiveness or practicality of it. It was for emergency lifesaving use only. I had the opportunity to use it only once, but the satisfaction I had from that procedure is worth more than what I paid for the very costly Storz (German) stiff bronchoscope, aa suction tip and the foreign body grasping forceps! Now, that bronchoscope is almost worthless (a museum piece, in fact). The latest ones are flexible and more sophisticated.

Remember the patient who was saved by the power of *japa*? Oe daye a relative of his came coughing to me. He was a regular betel nut and *beeda* chewer. He tossed a piece of betel nut up in the air, and aimed to catch it in his mouth. This dangerous practice is seen very frequently in villages – children toss toffees, groundnuts, and such things in the air, and aim to catch them in their mouth. Unfortunately, our man missed his aim and the betel nut piece fell into his throat, going right down his trachea. He coughed a lot but could not get it out. He waited for two days, but the piece was still stuck inside. His cough also became worse. He also developed a fever. That is when he came to consult me in Shimoga.

History itself was enough to diagnose a foreign body in the bronchial tree. Chest X-ray confirmed a collapse and patch of pneumonitis in the right base of chest. The betel nut piece had to be extracted as early as possible through a bronchoscope. The nearest places where this was possible were Bangalore and K. M. College, Manipal. He was not keen to go to either place though he could have afforded treatment at both those places. I explained to him that though I had a bronchoscope, I would have to use it under local anaesthesia, which is very, very uncomfortable to the patient. Besides I could not promise success, as this procedure actually needed a specialist and general anaesthesia. He refused to go anywhere else and promised to cooperate with me during the procedure. Seeing his relative come back from the jaws of death, he appeared to have more faith in me!

Dr Venn's teachings were about to be put to test. I used an atomiser to spray local anaesthetic into the throat. I made the patient lie on the operation table supine with his head hanging over the top end of the table. Then I gently manoeuvred the bronchoscope into his trachea and right bronchus. Luckily for me the betel nut piece was staring at me. It was lying where a bronchus was branching. I quickly grasped it and extracted it, when the patient gave a big cough to throw out some purulent material. I had been warned of such an event by Dr. Venn, and so I was well prepared for it. It sprayed over my facemask and the spectacles that protected my eyes. He was happy with the relief, and was very pleased. He was put on antibiotics and kept under observation for two or three days. He did not develop any complications, and went home. I was pleased with myself too.

"The reward of a thing well done is having done it."

- Ralph Waldo Emerson

My fees did not even cover a fraction of the cost of the bronchoscope, and I did not get another opportunity to use that bronchoscope again, right up to my retirement! Economics do not always make sense every time.

17. Urethral Stone: An Experiment That Succeeded

In rural practice, the approach to a surgical problem and its treatment must not only be effective but also affordable. Also, the end must justify the means. I am an old-timer now. Our teachings were very different; we were taught to make treatment affordable, to depend on clinical decisions as much as possible, to avoid costly investigations and to simplify procedures. Innovations were very helpful to reduce the costs. One well-known orthopaedic surgeon in the J. J. Group of Hospitals used to use wooden ice-cream spatulas as splints for fingers in hand surgery! Some patients were so poor that they could not afford even the medicine we prescribed, leave alone going for special investigations or specialists' care.

One such patient has stuck in my mind for more than 50 years. He was a teenaged boy from the neighbouring Navule village, a suburb of Shimoga; very poor and as a result, of sickly health, clear evidence of the pathetic poverty of the family. To top it all, he had a stone stuck in the external urethral meatus; it might have been formed and grown in the kidney higher up and somehow, painlessly slid down to the tip of his penis. He had difficulty emptying his urinary bladder every time, having to strain very hard to drive the urine out along the sides of the stone, and, needless to say, he had continuous pain. The urine stream was more like a spray! The tip of the calculus could be seen but it was not possible to grasp the calculus to pull it out. General anaesthesia would have been ideal to try and negotiate the calculus out; but we did not have any anaesthetist in town then, nor he could have afforded for his services if available. I could have given a local anaesthetic injection to make a small slit in the glans to extricate the stone. But he plainly refused any sort of interference. Besides, the boy was so poor that, even if I did the surgery free, he could not have even afforded the medicines that were going to be necessary after that surgery. So, in desperation, I advised him a very unorthodox treatment that one cannot find in any surgical book, and which would not cost him anything either. I asked him to climb up a stool and jump down, and to go on doing so, many times a day. I also wrote down a prescription for a few analgesic tablets. Anyone who heard me then would have concluded that I was out of mind and that my qualifications were fake. I would not have been surprised if they did. But I could not think of any other method to help him get relief.

To my utter surprise he came to me two days later to show the calculus that was like the seed of a palm date fruit! It fell down during one of his jumps! I laughed loudly and the boy could not understand why. Now it is perhaps the turn of the readers also to laugh at this madness. It could have been a coincidence, but I had not given up my belief that the jumping would help dislodge the stone.

Two to three years later, probably in 1973, a general medical practitioner's son from a neighbouring town Sirsi, some 140 km away came to me for consultation with an X-ray of his abdomen, which showed a calculus in the left ureter. He was a well-educated (in fact, an engineer), intelligent and very level-headed young man; he asked many questions on his problem and understood when I explained what I knew. He had abdominal pain due to the calculus being in the mid-section of his left ureter. After examining him and the X-ray, I told him that the stone was small and would likely pass out by itself. He said that he had waited for over two to three weeks and there was no change in the intensity or frequency of pain. That is why he had come this far, to find a quicker solution. We did not have a urologist who could have extracted that calculus by ureteroscopy and basketing! He would have had to go to a faraway hospital for this, and he was not ready for that. I told him to drink plenty of water every day, and hope to wash down the calculus.

"Is there any other method to hurry up the process?" he asked again. Then I told him that I knew of a very crazy method, which was not in any medical book. He could try it out if he wished to, but I could not promise him of any, let alone quick, results. He agreed, and I told him the story of the boy from Navule village, the how jumping down a stool repeatedly worked for him! He was amused but felt that there was some sense in the method. After all, do we not use similar manoeuvres to dislodge objects stuck in tubular passages like in bottle necks! He asked if he could ride a bicycle daily to and from his workshop. I told him that he certainly could, and also asked him to ride right through the potholes on the road so that he would get jolted very often! He went home brooding over my suggestion. I would not have been surprised if he felt a bit foolish about all this experimentation; but then, he had nothing to lose by trying!

A week later he rang me up to inform me that during one of the rides over a pothole, he felt a sudden pain in the abdomen, and the next day he passed the stone out in the urine. This could not be a coincidence too, could it?

My colleagues who heard about this method were very sceptic about it, and so I have not advised it to most patients who came to me with ureteric calculus. I did share it with a few who wished to know. But sadly, none came back to report the results. There are no double-blinded, multi-centric trials involving a large number of patients for this crude theory of mine, and so I do not venture to say that this is a method for universal prescription. Both cases could have been absolute coincidences, or as they say, the 'placebo effect'. However, can anyone say with confidence that the mechanical jerks could not have dislodged the stone downwards?

18. Ordinary Sugar for Infected Wound Dressings

Wound infection is a common occurrence in any surgical practice. Doctors use different materials to cover the wound or the ulcer with the hope that it may hasten the process of healing. Chemicals like silver nitrate, antiseptics and even antibiotics are used. But some ulcers and wounds refuse to heal.

My mother was a diabetic and she developed a foot infection that led to amputation. The amputation stump had a small sinus that refused to heal. I tried all tricks and all antibiotics and ointments but it did not heal. At such a time, my brother-in-law sent me a copy of a paper from an international competition for inventions/ innovations. It had entries from all over the world, in all fields like engineering, medicine, physics, and much more. This paper by Leon Herszage was about sugar dressings of surgical wounds.

I was tired of the chronicity of my mother's unhealed sinus. So, I decided to give sugar a try. I followed the paper and packed ordinary sugar, which we use for tea and coffee, raw so to say, into the sinus. In two days, when I changed the dressing, it was dry, and it remained so in the future! That encouraged me to use sugar for many other chronic wounds, and was happy to see encouraging outcomes.

Sugar and honey have been used from ancient times. The ancient Indian surgeon Sushruta (about 600 BC) used honey with ghee and a few other herbal ingredients to dress wounds. Similarly, ancient Egypt also used honey with lard to pack wounds. Although I do not know of any ancient records recommending sugar for wound dressing, it has been used in villages as a primary dressing for fresh wounds, for many years. Besides, it is cheaper than honey. Moreover, a scientific basis for it has also been established, with Herszage's paper.

Leon Herszage, a surgeon in Buenos Aires, Argentina, started using it in 1976, around the same time that Richard Knutson was using it in Greenville, Mississippi, USA. Both of them got good results. In 1980, Herszage and associates reported a cure rate of 99.2 percent after using sugar for wound healing in 120 patients.

His study revealed that:

1. Sugar in wounds does not get absorbed in the blood stream.

2. Sugar is hygroscopic and so it draws out the water from the plasma of bacteria, which therefore die. Sugar kills almost all organisms, even TB bacteria.

3. Hygroscopic effect also draws plasma from the blood vessels, into the wound, thus bringing with it the protective macrophages, enzymes, antibiotics used etc. I believe this phenomenon is very important.

4. Studies by others has shown that even if sugar is diluted to 50 percent by serum in the wound, it continues to be bactericidal.

5. Foul smell from the wound disappears in about a day or two.

The method of using sugar is quite simple. Just clean the wound as best as possible. Pour sugar (it does not need to be sterilised) or sugar paste (in water) on the wound or into the cavity of the wound to fill it up. Cover it with absorbent gauze and cotton and hold the dressing in place with bandage or tapes. Sugar in the wound may form a syrupy fluid and escape from under the dressings. Therefore, initially frequent change of dressing may be necessary. Otherwise, one daily change of dressing is adequate. One big problem is that ants get attracted to the patient's bed – this needs to be taken care of, and prevented as best as possible!

Sugar works like an antibiotic but without any of its side effects. However, it does cause some stinging discomfort to the patient. But since it is available so easily at such a low price, and since it is so effective, I preferred sugar over any other proprietary ointments, or honey, especially in very large wounds. More recent studies have revealed that sugar is even more effective if mixed with honey, which contains some enzymes; with hydrogen peroxide, especially for staphylococcal infections; with povidone iodine, which gives an additive effect, or poly-ethylene glycol.

I continued to use sugar for dressings to the end of my practice. I used to explain to the patient the problem of stinging when sugar is put on the wound and the likelihood of ants crawling to the wound site. But the effectiveness and very low cost were very strong convincing points. One diabetic lady had large subcutaneous abscesses over the abdomen, and over the back – a larger one stretching over half of the back area, and another small one near it. After draining the pus away, and with her consent, I started using sugar for dressings. It was impressive how soon the pus pouring out reduced and granulation tissue appeared on the wound. The diabetic status too became manageable. I taught her daughter the method of dressing those wounds and sent her home.

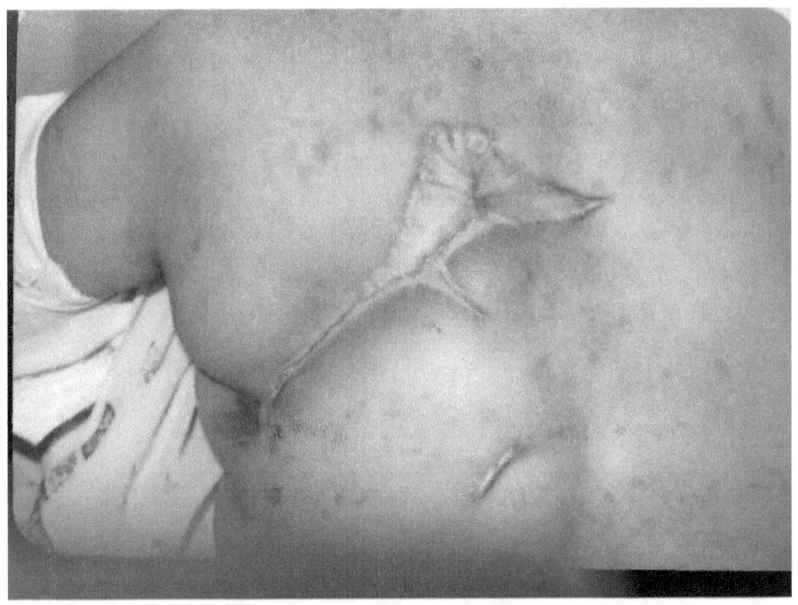

Figure 2: Scar of the sub-cutaneous abscess that had extended over three-quarters of the back area

Soon she came back with all the wounds healed. Had she used commercial ointments, she would have needed two to three tubes of ointment per dressing. Saving on the cost of these was substantial.

I have tried to popularise the use of sugar for dressings through various platforms. But, lack of interest amongst colleagues is surprising. Even a medical college looked at it with a closed, mocking mind. My nephew, who was a medical student, in Vadodara requested his Unit Head to try sugar in a very bad infected wound. He was told that he could do so if he wished but the seniors were not interested. He tried it diligently on his own and told me that the wound did get cleaner and less smelly, but main pathology was beyond his control!

We lack humility; we refuse to accept anything that is not Western or statistically-proved with double blinded studies, or recommended by the academic leaders.

Dr T. E. Udwadia from Mumbai is different. He did a study of honey (Sushruta's practice, circa 600 BC) for wound dressing and found it very effective. However, he felt that commercial honey available in India is adulterated and so, to be sure of the purity of the honey, he imported it from Australia for his series

!

19. Surgeries from Specialities

When I trained, there were only a few specialities. These were obstetrics and gynaecology, thoracic, Orthopaedics, neuro, cardiology, ophthalmology and ENT. General surgeons were taught and exposed to orthopaedics and urology, which were on the way to becoming specialties in their own right in the future. All general surgeons learnt the basics of most specialities. Perhaps that is why they were called 'General Surgeons'.

My work in Shimoga involved mainly abdominal surgery. But people in small towns and villages also develop specialty problems, and the nearest surgeon and even a general practitioner, has to treat them to the best of his capability. That is why I had to step into speciality areas. I treated thyroid, breast lumps, varicose veins, bones and joints, E.N.T. problems and so on, most of which have become specialities in their own right now! Just like my father, who, though a licentiate medical practitioner, had to often treat like an MBBS or even post graduate doctor, I too had to manage problems from higher specialities, if at all the patients were to be helped – as there were no specialists in Shimoga at that time. Later, even after specialists arrived in Shimoga, I continued treating some speciality cases, as and when needed. In the Royal College of Surgeons of Edinburgh in 1960s, the fellowship students were expected to know about almost all specialities! General surgery was truly general in those days. Many specialist problems may be seen only once in the rural surgeon's lifetime, like the case of the betel nut piece in a patient's bronchus; yet, they had to be managed, if the patient was to be helped.

Obstetrics & Gynaecology

In 1965, I had attended a course for the Fellowship of the Royal College of Surgeons of Edinburgh. Interestingly, RCSE believes that general surgery includes gynaecology and obstetrics. The syllabus included lectures by leading obstetrics and gynaecology teachers. I remember the joke by a lecturer on gynaecology; he asked us to tell the commonest cause for a rupture of the uterus, and a smart lady from the audience remarked loudly that it was the classical C-section performed by a general surgeon! Obviously, general surgery students must have been quite embarrassed. It revealed two truths to me: first, that general surgeons were being called upon to perform C-section deliveries; and, second, they needed to be trained to close the uterus properly. The inclusion of obstetrics and gynaecology in general surgery is perhaps true even today; About five years ago, I met a general surgeon from Shetland Hospital in Scotland. The hospital is situated in the sea far away from the shores of the main land. He confirmed that he was required to stand in for the obstetrician if she happened to be away, and even perform C-section deliveries, when the need arose. When I worked as a registrar in the UK, my 'boss' Mr Smith felt that jungle surgery must include obstetrics and gynaecology. So, he sent me to his colleague to expose me to this specialisation! He showed me the steps of a C-section surgery and hysterectomy, and shared some useful tips.

Later, in Shimoga, my wife started conducting deliveries and was gradually accepted as an obstetrician, although she is only an MBBS by qualification. I became her surgical arm in obstetrics. Suturing difficult episiotomies, performing C-section deliveries, and so on, were my responsibility. In gynaecology, the commonest surgery was hysterectomy. For a general surgeon that was not difficult to learn. I too learnt it from gynaecologists like my friend Dr Shirish Sheth and Dr Purandare from Mumbai, and Dr. Nagalaxmi in Shimoga who delivered our son. I also learnt vaginal salpingectomy for sterilisation (a family planning method) from Dr Shirish Sheth. So, in due course of time, I became quite adept at surgeries in this speciality. However, we avoided major surgeries involving extensive dissection and excision. Otherwise, our practice thrived quite well.

Orthopaedics

We studied orthopaedics as though it was a part of the general surgery syllabus. In our practice, fractures and dislocations were common occurrences. I had worked as a house surgeon in a busy orthopaedic and trauma unit, for surgeons like the well-known Dr Wayne Wright (Stoke-on-Trent, UK). In Shimoga, I treated most of the fractures that came to us in classical Charnley's closed reduction technique (that is, without resorting to surgery to introduce nails and plates to stabilise the fracture ends). But fracture of the neck of the femur eluded me. I had brought guide wires for use with Smith Peterson Pin to stabilise the femoral neck, but I could not use them, as I did not have any X-ray unit or C-arm in our OT. We treated such patients in a Thomas' splint, fabricated in a workshop in Shimoga. Children with femur fracture were treated in 'gallows' frame, again assembled in Shimoga. I had to manipulate and reduce a fracture blindly without the help of a C-arm unit. After each reduction of the fracture, the patient with POP cast had to be sent to the radiologist for a confirmation X-ray. I could not do plate and screw fixations of fractures, as these were not yet available in Shimoga, and there was difficulty with prolonged general anaesthesia. I also had to treat a couple of cases of osteomyelitis (infection of bones) in children. I followed the method given in the book at the time. I drained the pus, removed the dead bone, curetted the surrounding bone, packed the cavity with tincture Benzoin gauze, and then dressed and bandaged the limb. POP cast was then applied over it. Antibiotics were given. The wound was inspected periodically and fresh dressing and POP cast was applied. They took a long time to heal, but heal they did. One of them came back many years later, and I was happy to see that the bone, though not nice to see, had healed completely.

My aunt from Honnavar came to Shimoga one day with a swollen left elbow. She had fallen three days earlier and her children had ignored her complaint for reasons unknown. Even before I touched her, I knew that it was a 'neglected' (unattended by a doctor for a few days) elbow fracture. An X-ray revealed comminuted (multiple fragments) fracture of the lower end of humerus and upper end of ulna. Oedema was so severe that it looked like a balloon, and reducing the fracture was going to be difficult, and even dangerous. So, I chose to treat it by a method called a 'bag of bones'; that is, suspend the limb in a sling with a drip stand, until the oedema settles down. Then gradually flex the elbow in stages. When all the oedema disappeared, a POP back slab was applied in flexion position of the elbow. This method gave such wonderful results that it was difficult to say that she had such a bad fracture at all.

The son of a staff member had sustained fracture avulsion of the medial malleolus Rt. Ankle. It failed to heal even after long immobilisation. That made me think that probably a bit of periosteum was preventing the union. But we did not have any screws available in Shimoga. I got some from Bangalore. In my bone set (discards from the British hospital), was a usable hand drill and screw driver. When I exposed the fracture, a bit of periosteum was found to be interposed between the tibia and malleolar fragment. That periosteum was removed and the malleolus was fixed back in place with a screw. This time, the fracture healed.

My son came home on holidays in 1995, from his college in the US. He had fallen over snow a few days earlier. The emergency room in the hospital there had examined him with an X-ray of the wrist and told him that all was well. A bandage was wrapped on the wrist and he was sent home. At the airport, as he tried to lift his luggage, he suddenly winced. I noticed that, and on coming home, had his wrist X-rayed again only to find a scaphoid bone fracture. I promptly put the appropriate POP (Velcro) bandage, and he went back to the US with it. This bandage became a big topic of discussion in his US clinic, as they had advanced to fibre-glass casts without ever having seeing a Plaster of Paris one!

Accidents do happen in rural areas too, though they may not be road traffic accidents. Farm accidents also result in compound fractures and serious injuries. They can be attended to, in time, by a general surgeon to reduce morbidity and mortality. Despite the real need for orthopaedics in rural practice, I was surprised that even MS students are not exposed to orthopaedics in our medical colleges! I have written earlier about a Professor of Orthopaedics, who said "Why do you want to do orthopaedics at all? Send them all to us, we will manage!" How narrow-minded can someone be!

Paediatric Surgery

Here too, in the absence of specialised paediatric surgeons, I had to manage emergencies as best as I could. I had to manage obstructed or irreducible congenital inguinal hernias, undescended testes, intussusceptions, stomach obstruction of pyloric stenosis, and much more.

While talking about the successes, I am also reminded of an unsuccessful outcome. A paediatrician sent to me a boy with stomach outlet obstruction – congenital pyloric stenosis. These children vomit out all the milk drunk just then. Mild obstructions sometimes open up with medical treatment. But this was a severe obstruction. I had successfully released many such obstructions in the past. So, I operated on this boy too, and thought that I had done all that was needed. The boy recovered, healed well and went home. But he returned in a few days, vomiting again. Obviously, the release of the obstruction was not complete, which meant a repeat operation has to be done.

The paediatrician lost faith in my capability and sent the boy to Manipal for the second surgery. I never had any further referrals from that paediatrician in the future.

Parenteral infusion of fluids used to be a big problem for us in the early days. Scalp-vein sets, cannulas were not known as yet; so, we had to use injection needles to give IV fluids. When this failed, we had to infuse the fluids subcutaneously by injecting hyaluronidase in the area. Hyaluronidase increases the absorption of fluid in the area into the blood circulation but there was no way of monitoring the volume absorbed. Many a times, the last resort was to perform phlebotomy, that is, introduce a metal cannula or a plastic tube into the long vein at the ankle! Then came the scalp vein set, and even later, the capable paediatricians themselves.

Two babies stand out in my memory. Both had lumbar meningoceles. These new-borns were from nearby villages and the parents would not agree to go to proper higher centres like Bangalore or Manipal. Left to themselves, the meningoceles could rupture any time and then, the baby would not have much chances of survival.

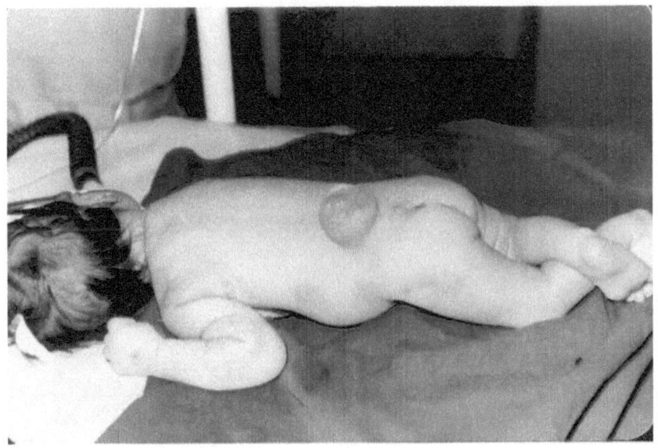

Figure 3: Lumbar meningocele in a baby

Both the babies (admitted at different times) were similar when we saw them. They were kicking their lower limbs, and did not show any spinal parts in the meningocele. The meningocele sacs were intact. Books said that the meningeal sac had to be excised as early as possible and a proper skin cover given to the defect. The paediatrician was not sure whether bladder and bowel control was normal. So, the choice before me was to perform the surgery and make a sincere attempt to save the babies. This was explained to the parents who wanted their baby saved but did not want to go to a faraway hospital.

I had my technical problems too. We did not have a paediatric anaesthetist, or the equipment for it. In desperation, we decided to use local anaesthesia supported by oxygen administered with a mask, by my wife, and gauze dipped in honey for the baby to suck on. Diluted lignocaine was used to anaesthetise the operation site. Slowly and patiently the sac was separated and then removed. The skin was closed and the surgery was over. In the other boy, the neck of the sac was an inch wide and the edges of the meninges had to be closed with the thinnest catgut sutures I had. Then the skin was closed.

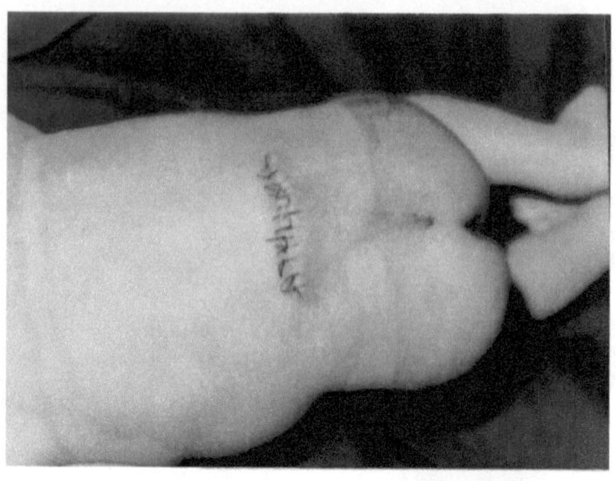

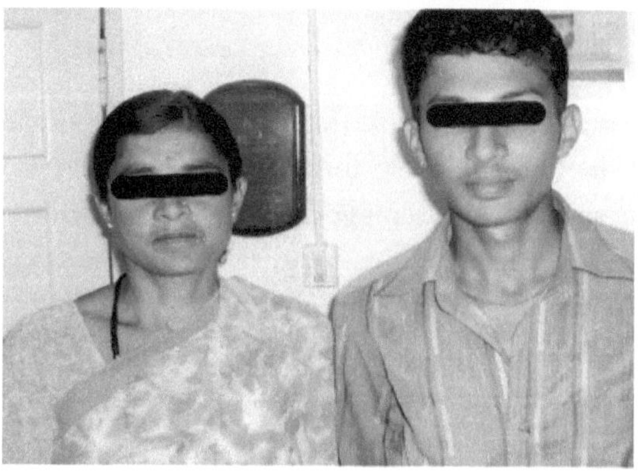

Figure 4: One of the boys operated for meningoceles, when he came for a follow-up 15 years later

Despite our cynicism and pessimism, both babies recovered well and went home. Around 15 years later one of them came to me for a follow-up check-up. I was happy to see a handsome young man walking into adulthood! His back was strong and straight, with a tell-tale scar. The only noticeable problem he had was a very slight limp on the left side.

Similarly, there was a baby with a sacro-coccygeal tumour. And the parents were not very keen to go to a bigger hospital. By this time, we too had an anaesthetist. So, we decided to perform the surgery in our small hospital.

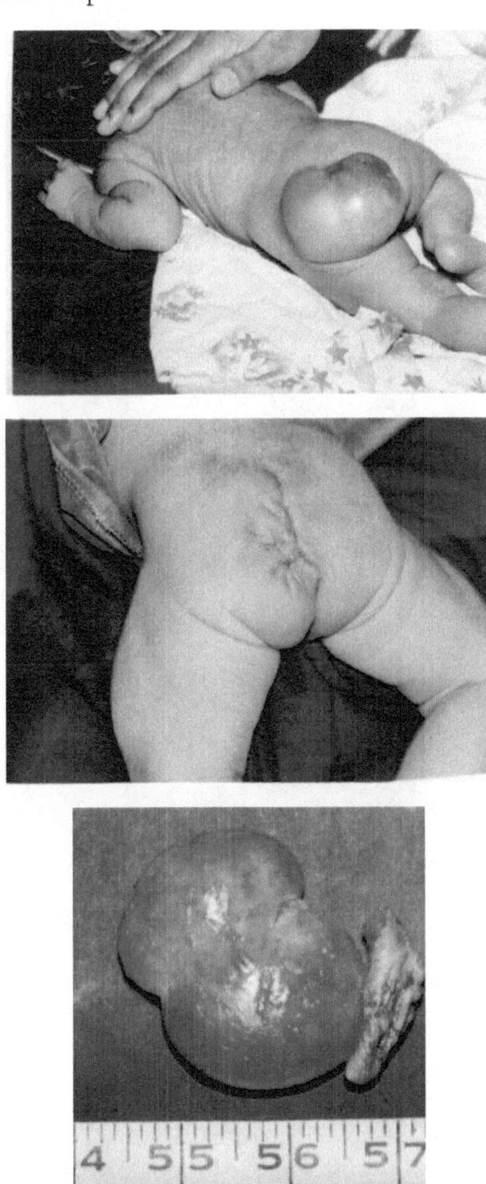

Figure 5: Sacrococcygeal tumour removed from a baby

Plastic Surgery

I have written about how I had the opportunity to work for a general surgeon who also performed plastic surgery. He was a first-batch student of Sir Harold Gillis. That encouraged me to bring back home some simple and basic plastic surgery instruments like fine skin hooks, small dermatome that used razor blade for a knife, and so on. I used these to remove a scar, rotate a flap to cover small raw areas, repair ear lobes, and so on.

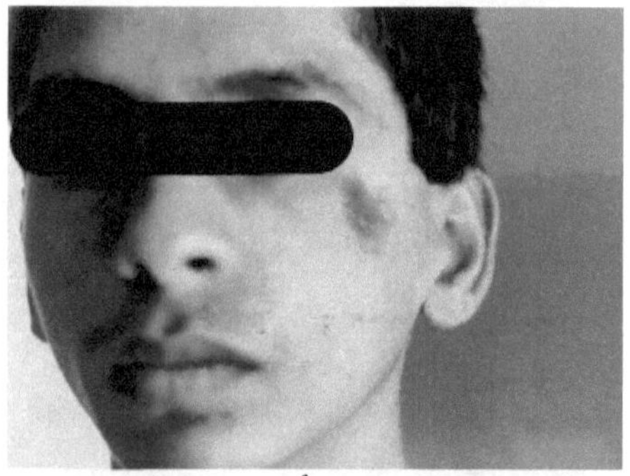

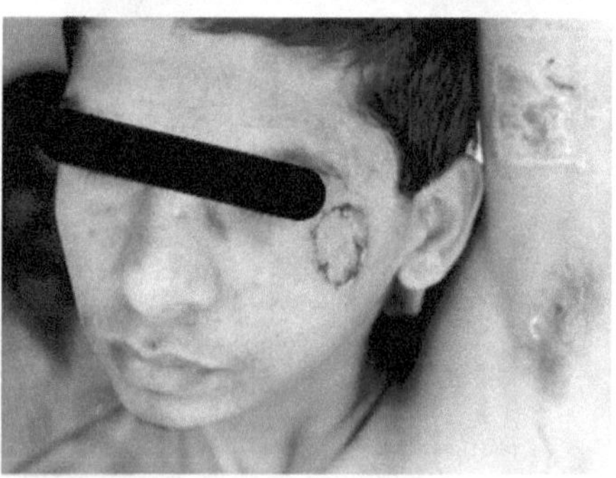

Figure 6: Removing a skin blemish on the left cheek of a boy

Once, a diabetic lady came with a large ulcer on the chin. I had read about grafting placental membrane on such ulcers, and with her consent applied it to her ulcer. Surprisingly, the membrane was not rejected and the ulcer healed in some days.

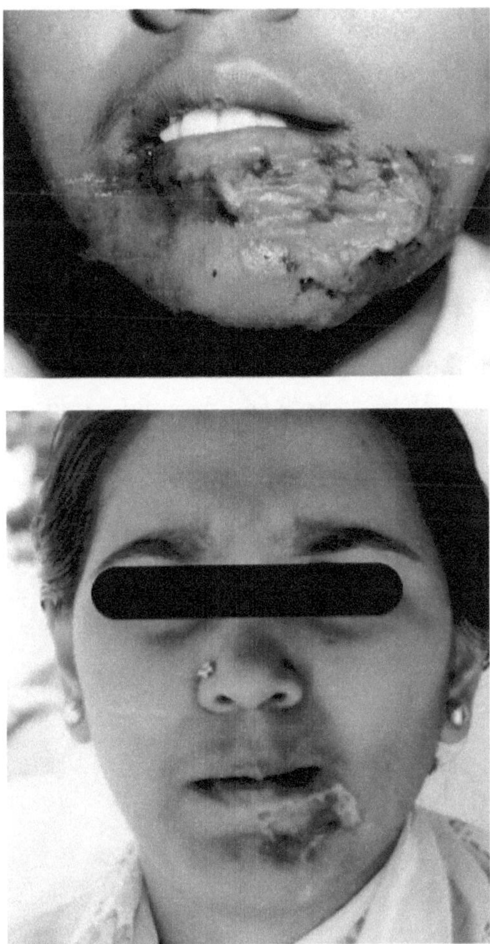

Figure 7: Healed by grafting placental membrane on the ulcer

Most of our post-treatment pictures were taken when the patients came for suture removal. Unfortunately, they hardly came for follow-up, when we could have had a picture of the healed dry surface!

One evening, a bigger problem presented itself to me. A boy was cleaning a rice mill, which had been switched off for that purpose. He was still up there working, when suddenly the mill came to life and the boy's pyjamas got caught in the mill. The pyjamas got twisted and pulled by the mill, and in the process, the boy's scrotal skin was avulsed. When I saw him, his penis and scrotum had been de-gloved, that is, did not have skin cover. I had never seen such a sight and also did not have a clue how to deal with it! My father-in-law, who loved surgery, and used to perform minor procedures too, had presented to me a copy of *Hamilton Bailey's Emergency Surgery*. I used to look into this book for tips on treatment of strange emergencies. I found the answer to this problem too! I had to clean the wound thoroughly, bury each testis in the subcutaneous tissue of the respective thigh on its side and then put a split skin graft from the thigh on the shaft of the penis. I could certainly do that. I was happy to see that the boy healed without any complications. Many years later he visited me. He was a man now, working in the Middle East, and to be married soon. He confirmed that everything was functioning normally.

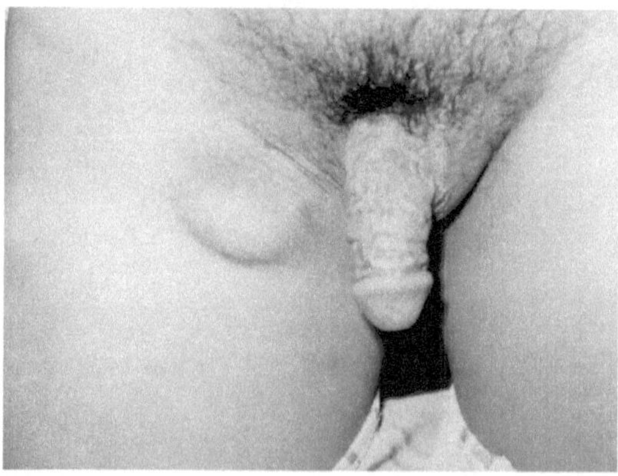

Figure 8: Treating a de-gloved penis and scrotum

I corrected a cleft lip too, under local anaesthesia. This was a poor girl, about ten to twelve years of age, who had a large wide cleft of the upper lip. Poverty kept her away from seeking surgical help. At that time, it was her grandmother who brought her to me as she was nearing a marriageable age. No amount of talking could convince her that she should go to a plastic surgery department. This was before the "smile train" programme. If I did not repair it, she would go home and nowhere else. Having seen and assisted in many repairs in the UK, I felt I could try and make a fair repair, but I did not have fine sutures, and none were available in Shimoga at the time. I used lignocaine infiltration anaesthesia and repaired the lip in proper layers. The end result was surprisingly very good. The grandmother had little to pay for the hospital and surgery cost. But the girl's happy smile was itself a satisfying payment. She too did not come back for a follow-up check! I hope she got married.

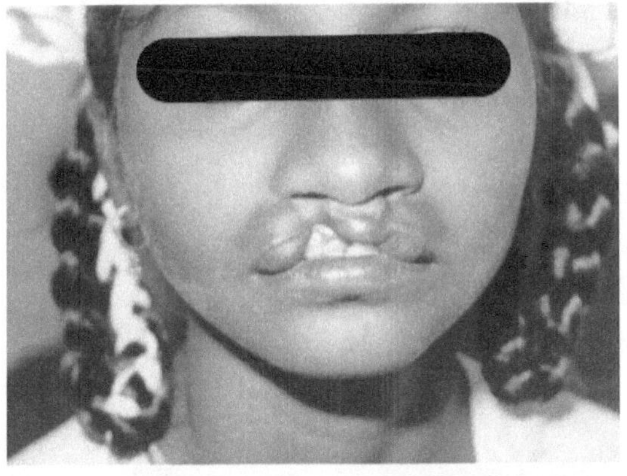

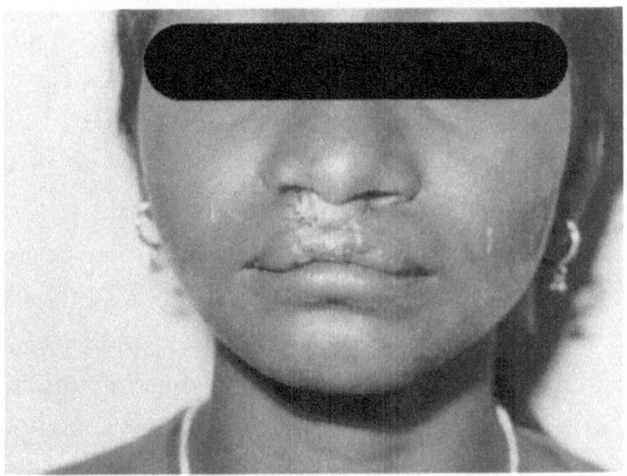

Figure 9: Repairing a large wide cleft of the upper lip

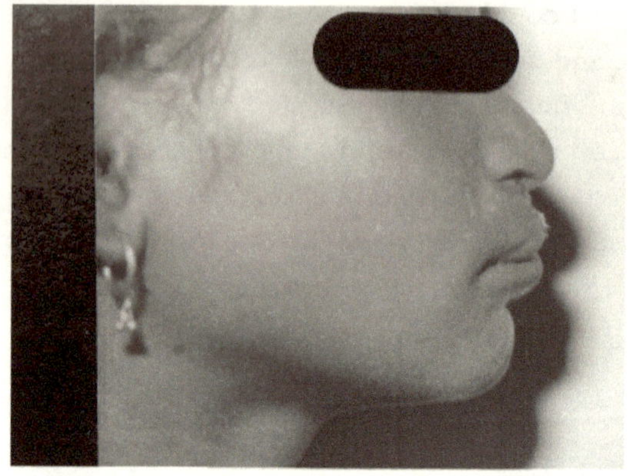

Figure 10(contd): Repairing a large wide cleft of the upper lip

Urology

My duties as a Resident Surgical Officer (RSO), during my last posting in the UK, involved working with a urologist also. Unfortunately, when I started the job, the urology consultant had retired and the job was unfilled. General surgeons treated urology patients (mainly benign hypertrophy of prostate), and preferred to refer only special problems to the urologist. The urologist was appointed rather too late for me to learn endoscopic prostate surgery from him. I had learnt cystoscopy (endoscopic inspection of urinary bladder) by then, and had even purchased a costly Ritchi's cystoscopy set to bring home to India. But I could not use it at all because of anaesthesia and blood transfusion difficulties. The additional time needed for cystoscopy made spinal anaesthesia unsuitable. On one occasion, when I did want to perform retrograde ureterography, the patient had to be carried to the radiologist half a mile away with the ureteric catheter in situ! So, I neither used the cystoscope set again, nor performed the Millin's (advanced and improved) retropubic prostatectomy that I was used to. Instead, I learnt the modified one-stage abdominal (Freyers) prostatectomy; another example that so-called old and obsolete surgical techniques were still relevant in rural surgery. Until a qualified urologist came to Shimoga, I had done quite a few prostatectomies by this old method, a few kidney stones and bladder stones surgeries, and such.

ENT

Having a foreign qualification (FRCS) attracted patients from almost all surgical specialities to me. Having worked with different specialists in different hospitals in the UK was just as well. It gave me confidence to treat many patients. Many ENT patients came in, and I ventured to do some tonsillectomies too. I had to drain one with Ludwig Angina (abscess in the floor of the mouth) and a one with Quincy (abscess in tonsillar area). I had to remove foreign bodies from noses, throat and ears too. One patient had a fish bone stuck in his throat while eating in an inebriated state. Another patient stands out in my memory. He reminded me that old ayurvedic methods are still viable and useful.

A boy came from the neighbouring district, complaining of a bad smell in his nose. In fact, one could not go near him because of it. On examination, I found out that he had Rhinitis sicca; in this the nasal cavity dries up and the mucus in the whole nasal cavity too dries up into 'plaques 'or 'flakes' that line the inner surface of the nose. Mucus under these plaques decomposes, and gives out an awfully bad smell. The patient develops severe halitosis. In those days, I could not find any easy treatment for this. The only solution was to get all those dried mucus plaques out and to 'wash' the nasal cavity daily. My father was with me. He suggested that Magnesium Sulphate in Glycerine, sometimes help. This was not a proprietary preparation and there were no dispensing chemists in those days. So, I prepared a thick solution of Magsulph powder in Glycerine and gave it to the boy and asked him to use it as drops in to the nose twice a day; evening drops to be instilled before going to bed. I also told him about a yogic practice of cleaning nose; I think it is called *jala neti*. It involves pouring water in one nostril with a spouted pot and letting it out from the other, and repeating the process from the other nostril. This not only washes the nasal cavity, it keeps it wet too. Using plain water causes severe discomfort in the nose. So, it is usually advised to use normal saline in initial stages and then gradually switch over to water.

The boy came after a month or so. Magsulph solution was over in a few days and he was now practicing the *jala neti* every day. And he was very happy with the results. His nose was never as clean as now. I examined the nose and yes, it was clean and without a foul smell.

20. A Simple Rectal Digital Examination Saves a Patient

Clinical examination as such is dying. Everyone wants a lab report or a gadget to diagnose almost every disease, even before, or instead of touching a patient! Unfortunately, there are gadgets available for the different human functions too. This was revealed to me very clearly recently, when I asked a ward nurse in a hospital what the patient's pulse rate was. She ran and came back with a small digital pulse-oximeter to apply to the patient's finger to count the pulse rate. I was appalled and amused at the time. Maybe I am old-fashioned, but I do believe that a proper elicitation of history from a patient, a simple clinical examination and holding the wrist to feel the different characters of the pulse go a long way in arriving at a correct diagnosis. By not holding a patient's hand and feeling the pulse, a doctor is bound to miss noticing missed beats, low volume pulse beats, extra-systoles condition of the arterial wall, and such things. The simple act of touching and holding a patient's hand instils confidence in the patient also.

There are some things that we must not try to bypass. For example, asking patients about their daily health functions. These are indicators of the vital activities of the patient. I remember from my student days; in a surgical ward in the J. J. Group of hospitals, there was an Anglo-Indian ward sister who was unpopular because of her regimentations in the ward. But she always managed to win the 'Best Kept Ward' award year after year because of her military-like discipline in the ward. During her morning rounds in the ward with the staff nurse in charge, there were four questions that she would ask every patient (I know it because I was a patient in her ward!), in her twisted Bombay Hindi: "*Soya kya?*" (Did you sleep well?), "*Pishab kiya?*" (Have you emptied your bladder?), "*Sundas hogaya?*" (Had bowels opened?), and "*Khana khaya kya?*" (Have you had breakfast?) I feel doctors too must make a habit of asking questions like this. Each of those questions indicates a particular aspect of the progress or deterioration of the patient in the ward. I am generally against making anything a "routine" practice, but these questions are vital. In our intense involvement in checking the reports and charts, we tend to forget to converse or even have human contact with the patient, and so, we miss out such basic functional information, which is an indicator of good health.

Old teachers tried to drive in the importance of such approaches with aphorisms (for per rectal digital examination) like: *'If you don't put your finger in to it, you will put your foot into it!'* that is to say that you will miss some very important finding.

Most of us do not take that seriously. But a thorough clinical examination can save a patient, as in this case. A per rectal/ digital rectal examination (PR/ DRE), which forms a part of clinical examination in some cases, is shunned by most as it is 'dirty', and is even avoided by many surgeons. I remember a physician consultant (Professor of Medicine) sending me a note saying: "Come and do a PR examination on my patient." This examination could be very revealing and informative, and even life-saving! An interesting thing happened in my life that showed how one such small lapse can create disastrous complications.

Around 30 years ago, my uncle, an elderly man, had some medical problems like hypertension, diabetes and some cardiac condition. His own son was a general practitioner with an MBBS.

The patient needed to be hospitalised and he was, naturally, shifted to the care of the professors who had taught, and were highly respected by, the doctor son. All the tests and investigations were done, and all the standard and proper medications were given. But unfortunately, the patient did not improve; and instead, was getting worse. They did many more tests and tried many other types of medications, without success. The patient was tired of their care and wanted to go home. His wife was telling them repeatedly that the patient had not had his bowels open. The doctors probably tried all the usual medical measures, disposable enemas without assessing the situation properly. In any case, the patient's wife was not at all satisfied with the results. The patient became confused, and then semi-comatose. Having given up the practice of performing a DRE, the professors probably did not even think about the possibility of constipation being the root cause of the trouble. As the adage goes: *"Eyes do not see what the mind does not know!"*

Considering the patient's cardiac condition, and given that he was not responding to their standard medication, the professors felt there was nothing more for them to do, and advised the son to take the patient home, to be with his near and dear ones in his last days.

The patient's wife, my aunt, had a request for her son. She wanted to give one last try in Shimoga (my place). My cousin rang me up, and said he was bringing his father to Shimoga at his mother's wish for convalescing, but he slyly avoided telling me about his father's serious health status! I said I was only too happy to have them, thinking that my medical colleagues would be able to help him in his cardiovascular condition.

But when they arrived, I was in for a big surprise, nay a shock. Normally, my uncle was a huge person, over 6-foot tall, and heavily built. But the person who was brought in from an ambulance, on a stretcher, was a wasted, unmoving and semi-comatose body. I was speechless for some time, but I was committed to my invitation.

So, I took him in wondering about our next moves. The scanty notes, more like a list of drugs, did not help me much about his true status. The list of investigations and medication was impressive, but as is common nowadays, there were no notes about a proper diagnosis, the prognosis or follow-up advice.

His wife (intelligent but not literate) was in tears about her whole experience in the hospital (nursing home) up till that day. The doctors came and went everyday but hardly ever talked to her. She wanted to talk to them, but never got a chance. Her husband was gradually deteriorating. He had not passed stools for many days and that was bothering her naive mind; and despite her telling it, no one took a serious note of it.

When I went near the patient, there was a distinct tell-tale fetor. He was semi-comatose, or maybe even comatose. His limbs were flail, abdomen though not distended, was full. Blood pressure and other parameters were routinely recorded. Then I decided to do a digital rectal examination. The rectum was packed with hard dry faeces. It was so hard and tight that my finger could not go in very far. Immediate evacuation was imperative. So, I began removing the hard faeces (scybala) digitally as much as I could (the process is described as 'digital evacuation of faeces'), and even more was found to be there above. We tried a small surgical enema with soap and water, but the patient could not retain the fluid and it just came out. We made a second attempt for digital evacuation, and by then some more faeces had descended down; a lot more faeces came out. Higher faeces were softer. The enema was repeated and some faeces escaped with the water. Digital evacuation and enema were repeated quite a few times. The patient was in no condition to resist or complain of pain during all this, even though some rectal bleeding also occurred. But the sight of large masses of faeces escaping out was encouraging. Later enemas were far more successful in driving out semisolid and then semiliquid material from the colon. By then, the whole room had a faecal odour but I was happy that the colon was now getting rid of faeces. The enema (we were using soap and water for enema) was repeated a couple of times over the next few days till we found by digital examination that the rectum and colon were fairly empty.

Literature advises saline enemas, glycerine enemas to soften the stools, plain tap water enema and even bisacodyl enemas to stimulate the colon.

Since there was little else to be done for his hypertension or cardia, we continued the administration of the drugs advised by the physicians, along with simple nursing and a good nutritious diet. I started him on Milk of Magnesia and Isabgol (psyllium husk) on a daily basis. His wife's loving care, homely food of his liking, and rest was all we could offer him. After a week or so, he started eating properly and bananas were added to his diet. No other special treatment was given. There was no appreciable change in the first few days. After a week or ten days of his arrival in Shimoga, one morning he opened his eyes and asked his wife, "Where are we?" in a most touching, cinematic way. All of us were very thrilled with his getting out of the semi-comatose state. He was still weak and not fully-orientated but was awake and identifying us.

From then onwards, it was one happy story of continuous improvement in his mental status, health, food intake and physical activities. His taste and appetite improved and he enjoyed his food. We had to resort to some other stool softeners and laxatives to keep the bowel evacuated. Soon he started walking with help, and then all by himself. *Gokulashtami* (Lord Krishna's birthday) festival arrived and it was a pleasant sight to see him sit through the whole *puja* and conduct an *aarti* by himself. Finally, one day he felt he was strong enough to go back home. After a tearful farewell to us, he went home to live for a few years more! His was a most heart touching and satisfactory recovery for me and our family. I truly believe that if only any one of his earlier doctors had put a finger up his rectum, they might not have decided to write him off as they did.

This is becoming a common problem with the ageing population. Patients are weak, mostly bedridden, with associated medical conditions and often depressed; all these conditions lead up to bad bowel habits and constipation.

I have seen more such patients, all of whom recovered dramatically after a good colonic 'washout'. The latest was an 80-year-old lady with a benign pancreatic tumour, and multiple other medical problems, including some vague mucosal atrophy that had hindered her food choice, quantity and frequency for over 15 years. Because of her knee arthritis and operated hip fracture, her mobility was limited. Because of limited mobility and dislike of activity, there was muscular wasting. Lack of activity, poor food intake and absence of fibre in food gradually led to irregular bowel habits, incomplete evacuation, and so on, finally leading to constipation. Simple laxatives were not effective. She complained of desire to pass stools all the time, but inability to do so; a feeling of incomplete evacuation even when she passed liquid stools. A few days earlier, her abdomen had given me an impression that the pancreatic tumour had spread to the liver, which felt knobbly! But retrospectively thinking, all this was in fact a transverse colon loaded with 'hard' faeces. She became morose, had a bitter taste in the mouth and dislike for food, bad smell and lack of interest in the surroundings and visitors! We felt she may not last very much longer. Here again, digital examination revealed the impacted faeces in the rectum, and we had to resort to repeated evacuation of rectum with digital removals and simple soap and water enema to expel a surprisingly large quantity of faeces. She passed masses of stools over the next two days. In a few days after this, she became lively, liked her food, and started taking an interest in her own affairs. She even agreed to start making attempts to walk!

Even some medications including narcotics, too much of coffee, alcohol, and diseases like diverticulitis, endocrine disorders and psychogenic disorders may induce constipation. The colon can hold about a kilogram or more of stools; but in the case of constipation, it may contain 5 to 8 kg! Prolonged constipation itself becomes a disease that debilitates the patient. The intestinal bacterial toxins get absorbed into the blood and affect the different systems, like the brain, liver, kidney etc. adversely, though I have not found many references in this regard. There is a balance between beneficial and harmful bacteria in the gut, a state which the Russian-French zoologist Élie Metchnikoff termed as orthobiosis. Orthobiosis is said to enhance health, and delay senility. Poor health and irrational use of antibiotics destroys this delicate balance of bacteria in the gut and the unhealthy bacteria, yeast and parasites dominate. This is called dysbacteriosis (dysbiosis), that is, a microbial imbalance or maladaptation.

Inside the body, the mucosa of the gut normally prevents entry of bacteria into the circulation. In constipation, the mucosa is damaged and harmful bacteria enter the blood stream. In extreme cases, this may lead to death. The toxins in the gut and colonic gases including methane and hydrogen sulphide are absorbed into the blood and excreted through lungs and sweat giving that characteristic nasty faecal odour to breath and sweat. However, the treatment is simple; it is just evacuation of the rectum and colon. The end result is most satisfying.

Nowadays it is easier as medicines can do that. But first, clinicians must be ready to put their finger up the rectum of their patient!

21. Association of Rural Surgeons (ARSI) and More

In the early days of my practice I struggled to gather information on how to practice western (high income country) surgical practice in our low income country. I tried to find information and guidance to solve the difficulties faced by me in my practice, and information on the requirements of a small hospital, from the Association of Surgeons of India (ASI). They did not have any information, nor were they interested in that direction either. I tried to contact presidents of ASI, professors and senior surgeons but none could/would help. Most of them did not have the remotest understanding of what rural practice meant or a rural surgeon's difficulties. In 1986-87, I was Chairman of the Karnataka State Chapter of ASI (KSC of ASI had decided to have rural surgeons on its board), and Professor N Rangabashyam, the President of ASI in office was the chief guest for the state chapter conference. He was surprised that I, with a double FRCS, had decided to settle in Shimoga, while I could have earned multiple times that either in Bangalore or Chennai! Then I discussed with him the difficulties faced by surgeons like me, who practiced in rural areas. He did not have any clue about these, or about rural surgery. Unlike all the other top surgeons that I had met, Dr N Rangabashyam was the first surgeon who was humble and honest enough to confess that he did not know about our difficulties and was generous enough to think that the ASI ought to help these members too. The concept of rural surgery had found acceptance and a foothold in the ASI when he formed the Rural Health Care Committee (RHCC), with me as its Chairman. In 1988, the committee wanted to conduct a useful survey of rural surgeons amongst all the members of the ASI, and the biased and uncooperative ASI Secretary had to be reminded by Dr T E Udwadia (the President then) that survey was the work of the ASI, and so ASI has to fund it and conduct it. The survey was an eye opener:

- 96 percent performed abdominal surgery

- 80 percent performed obstetrics and gynaecology practice

- 68.3 percent performed orthopaedic surgery, and

- 66 percent practiced urology.

Obviously, most of the rural surgeons were multi-speciality practitioners. They were all interested in learning skills from other specialities; now even WHO has prepared a list of 44 essential skills required in rural surgery, that include those from most other specialities! So, the RHCC tried to fulfil their demands; it organized separate sessions for rural surgeons during the annual conferences of the ASI, the ASICONs. ASI did not allot any funds for this; RHCC was directed to bear all the expenses including travel expenses of the invited speakers! Famous personalities spoke at the conferences. Dr Purandare (obstetrics and gynaecology) gave a lecture on C-section delivery by a rural surgeon, in a meeting of rural surgeons in an ASICON in Indore! The lecture hall was jam-packed, which showed how much general surgeons were interested in an obstetric subject. Dr Balu Sankaran, retired Director General of Health Services, Government of India, came by himself to ASICON in Hyderabad and spoke about surgery in district hospitals, which is also rural surgery in essence. All this was so popular that there was a huge demand for a separate section of ASI for rural surgeons, so that they may then organise programmes that they are interested in. ASI refused to sanction it.

Dr T. E. Udwadia, while in office as the President of the ASI (1988), and at other times too, was the only other ASI president who supported rural surgery whole-heartedly. He even included rural surgery in the prestigious golden jubilee seminar in 1988 on "Appropriate technology in surgery in India by 2000 AD." I was asked to talk about Rural surgery. I had said at the time that our medical education and training at the time, was more suitable to those wishing to work in UK, and that we need to make suitable changes in the curriculum to suit our country and our people. The same view is echoed now, 32 years later, by Dr. Vikram Patel, Pershing Square Professor of Global Health and Wellcome Trust Principal Research Fellow at Harvard Medical School (USA), in an interview in the weekly "The Week" in August 2023! Later, when Dr. Udwadia became the editor of the Indian Journal of Surgery (IJS), he published a special issue of IJS wholly devoted to rural surgery! All this shows the faith Dr Udwadia had in rural surgery and in its role in healthcare in India. But the other succeeding ASI presidents were only condescending towards rural surgeons, without any concrete plans to help. Serious rural surgeons were upset with the ASI's refusal to sanction it a section, and they decided to break away from ASI and form their own independent association - the Association of Rural Surgeons of India (ARSI).

The important founding team that met in Shimoga in 1992 and decided to form the ARSI, included Dr Balu Sankaran, Ex DGHS, Professor of Orthopaedics, St. Stephens College, Delhi, advisor for WHO etc. Dr N. H. Antia (retired Professor of Plastic Surgery, J. J. Group of Hospitals, and advisor to the Government of India on health policies), Dr J. K. Banerjee (Delhi), Dr R. R. Tongaonkar and Dr Asha Tongaonkar (Dondaicha, Maharashtra), Dr B Venkata Rao, my wife and myself from Shimoga and Dr.

R.P.Pai Manipal. The expenses for this meeting were borne by Dr. J.K.Banerjee from funds he had received for his dream rural hospital in Delhi. Later, many important practicing rural surgeons, who supported the idea forming the ARSI joined hands with us, like Dr Shipra Banerjee, Dr Sitanath De, Dr K. C. Sharma, Dr Sivasubramaniam and Dr Dakshinamurthy.

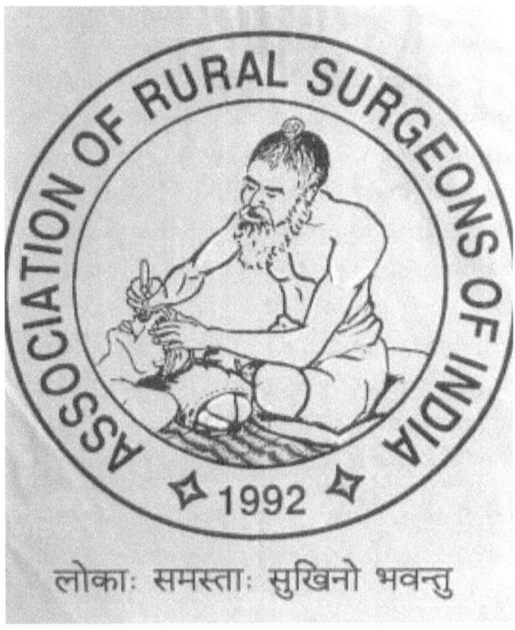

Figure 11: ARSI's Logo and Motto

ARSI was launched at the Mahatma Gandhi Institute of Medical Sciences, at Wardha, during its first conference there, in 1993. Later a large number of enthusiastic rural surgeons from all over India had gathered to launch this association. The elderly Dr Ramamurthy came with a group from Kanchipuram, Dr Brahma Reddy came with his hospital team from the then, Andhra Pradesh. Dr K. C. Sharma came from Jammu. Everyone hailed it and we felt happy too. The membership was, and is open to many types of medical graduates, obstetricians, anaesthetists, and so on. After an initial surge in membership, it slowed down. I was its Secretary for the first eight years, then President for two years. ARSI encourages innovations that will be useful in rural surgery; one such innovation has now become popular worldwide – the mosquito net for hernia repair. ARSI is currently supporting the fight for legalising Unbanked Direct Blood Transfusion (UDBT).

After about thirty years, I am convinced that we did the right thing to form our own ARSI. We could not have achieved what we have achieved if we were a part of the ASI. In these past 30 odd years I have found that the ASI, nor its successive presidents have ever tried to understand rural surgery or about the changes needed to take appropriate, affordable health care to the last person in the country. Interactions with prospective and in office presidents revealed that they are not interested in that topic at all. Unfortunately, the government too has more interest in the proliferating corporate hospitals and tertiary hospitals rather than improving the primary and secondary care hospitals.

It is interesting to note that western (developed) countries have realised the importance of rural physicians for their own countries and have started training programmes for them to face the difficulties and peculiarities of their rural areas. USA has at least fourteen such programmes. Scotland had Remote and Rural surgery training programme, Australia and New Zealand too have their own programmes. But, and it is a shame that Bharat that is India has none of such programmes. Sadly, and it is a shame again, that medical colleges including those that call themselves rural medical colleges, and professors who should have taken a lead in such training were/are in the forefront to object to every effort made by ARSI, IGNOU and Board of Examinations to impart such training. Despite all the hurdles and disappointments, ARSI has gone ahead with its own programmes in various fields.

To empower rural surgeons, ARSI had conceived the idea of training rural surgeons by 'distant education' with the help of the Indira Gandhi National Open University (IGNOU). We all put our ideas together and prepared a course for a Certificate in Rural Surgery (CRS) under the guidance of Dr. T.K.Jena of IGNOU. But only the Mahatma Gandhi Memorial Institute of Medical Sciences came forward to take it up. All other medical colleges refused. Even when the National Board of Examinations tried to revive it as DNB in Rural Surgery, it failed to attract medical colleges, mainly because they were not interested in it. So, it was dropped.

On its own, the ARSI encouraged its members to learn newer technologies by offering some financial assistance (Shimoga-Jhargram scholarship). Many members learnt ultra-sonography, laparoscopy, upper GI endoscopy, and so on. Many workshops were organised, free of charges, to encourage members to learn new surgical techniques, simple plastic surgery procedures, simple paediatric procedures, etc. But there was a severe fund crunch!

In big metropolises, the poor patients are similar to rural patients. In Delhi, to reach the poor patients, Dr J. K. Banerjee, Dr Shipra Banerjee, and their colleagues like Dr Basu, Dr Toor and others built a Rural Medicare Centre in Mehrauli (near the Qutb Minar) to offer affordable healthcare to everyone. Dr Banerjee and his wife, Dr Shipra, put in a lot of efforts in the initial stages of the evolution of rural surgery in India and in the formation of the ARSI.

One of our association members, Dr Brahma Reddy, introduced the idea of using a commercial mosquito net for the repair of inguinal hernia way back in 1994 during the second conference of the ARSI. Dr R. R. Tongaonkar popularised it, and wrote about it in the special edition of the IJS that was devoted to rural surgery. Professors of surgery raised many questions about lack of controlled trials, no animal experiments with the mosquito mesh etc. etc. Dr. Udwadia rightly pointed out to them that they have the means and resources for all that and so they must do all that work! I do not think they did that either. Dr. Tongaonkar's work attracted attention worldwide, and he was even invited to present a paper at a global forum in Dubai where someone remarked that developed countries too should be using it. But our own professors were, and are sceptical about it ven now! Dr Tongaonkar supplied the net in bulk, free of cost, to African surgeons. Thousands of African patients were benefited by this. Dr Tongaonkar also worked very hard to get a government sanction for the use of UDBT.

The use of carbon dioxide for laparoscopic surgery has its own setbacks. So, some Indian surgeons started using air instead and found that there were no problems. Then someone found a way to increase intra-abdominal space by lifting the abdominal wall up instead of distending the abdomen with gas or air. This Indian 'laparo-lift' technique became popular and our member Dr Gnanaraj, who went on to become President of the ARSI and is currently the Secretary of the International Federation of Rural Surgery (IFRS). He refined and popularised it under the name of Gas Insufflation Less Laparoscopic Surgery (GILLS). He even conducted workshops to train those interested in it. Dr Gnanaraj's efforts have resulted in the following:

- Gas Insufflation Less Laparoscopic Surgeries

- The ARSI's memorandum of understanding (MoU) with the Martin Luther King University, for short and specific courses for rural surgeons, like "Spinal Anaesthesia for Medical Officers and Rural Urology Practice," and

- The lap-top cystoscope and rural urology.

Dr Gabriele Holoch and Dr Peter Thomas of the German Society for Tropical Surgery (DTC) noticed the activities of the ARSI. They even invited me, to address and tell its members the activities of ARSI during their annual conferences in Munich, Germany. African delegates that had attended that conference became interested in

ARI philosophy. Later some African surgeons and rural surgeons from USA started participating in our annual conferences. Dr J. K. Banerjee had attended a conference in South America, where our concept of rural surgery was greeted with cheers by the delegates.

Though the concept of rural surgery may vary from country to country, the basic principles are the same, i.e., reaching the unreached. All this led to the proposal by Dr Thomas of DTC, for an International Federation of Rural Surgery (IFRS). During the ARSICON in Ujjain (2005) it was unanimously accepted, and the IFRS was duly launched during that conference. Rural surgery concept is very popular in Africa, and the IFRS spread there fast. Surgeons from India, U.S.A, Tanzania, Germany, Holland, Uganda and Kenya were signatories to the memorandum.

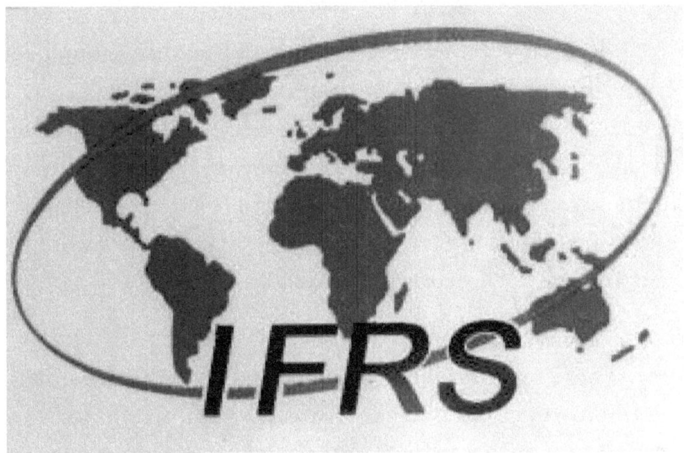

Figure 12: The International Federation of Rural Surgery was formed in 2005

Dr Pascience Kibatala from Tanzania was an active overseas member of the ARSI. He was successful in establishing rural surgery in his country. He organised a conference of the IFRS in Tanzania in 2007. We are sorry to have lost him.

Dr Oluyombo Awojobi (popularly Yombo) from Eruva Nigeria was a dynamic, dedicated rural surgeon. He started a rural surgeons' association in Nigeria (ARSPON), became secretary of the IFRS, and demonstrated innovative skills during his practice. He developed a mechanical centrifuge with an old bicycle frame using sound physics principles! Not having a good road in his area, he created an ambulance on a motorcycle. He even organised an IFRS conference in Nigeria in 2011. We are sorry to have lost him too, a few years later.

ARSI has been planning and working primarily for rural India. This philosophy and work of the ARSI attracted the attention of Lancet Global Health. ARSI is now a partner with Lancet Global Health in its project of Global Surgery by 2030.

I am very happy that rural surgery has now become recognised by its own good work and efforts, that it has its own independent association, and has spread beyond the national borders to faraway countries. I am happy that the ARSI was bold enough to be the first to accept the use of mosquito nets in hernia repair, when professors had rejected it. The ARSI even awarded a prize for this innovation. Now it is accepted worldwide.

But the sad thing is that the membership of ARSI is not growing. There must be thousands of rural surgeons in India, who are still not members of the ARSI. ARSI does not seem to have any schemes to attract them; I am also not aware of any incentives or assistance offered by the Health Department to promote rural surgery. ARSI and the Government must work together, and think about this seriously. I believe that rural surgery, or global surgery, is more relevant for India in the future.

22. Some Bold Decisions and Some Disappointments

As in anyone's life and career, I too made some bold decisions I am proud of, as also some disappointments still lingering in my memory.

Operating on close relatives

It is a common accepted practice not to perform surgery on one's close relatives, though it is not illegal. There may be various reason for and against it, but it all depends upon the particular case in hand. William Osler recommended over a century ago that surgeons require detachment and imperturbability because the permanence of major surgery is counterintuitive.

I have had to operate on my close relatives on more than one occasion. On looking back, they were bold decisions. They were uncomplicated surgeries of necessity and urgency. Fortunately, all those who underwent these surgeries healed well. But operating on my own father was a totally different matter!

I landed in a very delicate situation when my father, at the age of 89, developed urinary retention. I was away at that time in Bangalore, for an ASI Conference. By the time I returned home the next day, a suprapubic catheter had been inserted by a colleague of mine. Obviously, the prostate was pretty large, as confirmed by digital examination and an ultra-sonograph; ultra-sonography had arrived in Shimoga by then. I was happy that we had a qualified and capable urologist in Shimoga. However, when we had the preoperative assessment done by a physician and a cardiologist, we were shocked, because they unhesitatingly declared my father unfit for the surgery. He had had two MIs in the past, there was an aneurysm of left ventricle, and in that, there was a large ball like clot, ejection fraction was around 30 percent, and so on. The leading anaesthetist in town refused to anaesthetise my father. The urologists said that my father needed prostatectomy; trans-urethral resection is a prolonged procedure, unsuitable in view of his cardiac condition. He needed a quick-in and quick-out Freyer's supra-pubic enucleation. But he was not ready to do it!

I discussed with the alternatives with my father; he could either choose to live with a catheter for the rest of his life, and that may mean a poor quality of life with infection and uriniferous smell around him all the time, or we could risk a surgery, which may be very dangerous. He asked for my personal opinion, and I told him my honest belief that surgery despite the risk would be my choice. Then he gave his decision. He was ready to undergo surgery, provided that one, I – and only I – perform the surgery, and two, that the surgery was performed in our own nursing home! If I was not willing to do it, he would rather live with the catheter. His trust in my surgical skills was total but scaring for me. He had often complimented me in the past saying that he had not seen such 'clean' surgeries before. So, he decided to submit himself to my scalpel! Now I had to take the final call. I could not bear to imagine my father walking around with a urine bag in one hand and urine smell wherever he went. My choice was surgery and I had to perform it, just like the spinal anaesthesia I had to give to my wife at the start of our practice!

I decided to consult my mother and told her about need of the surgery. She did not worry at all. She had uncontrolled diabetes, which had resulted in bilateral leg amputations and delicate health. But father's cardiac status was far more precarious. She believed that it did not matter much. Our astrologer had assured her long ago that my father would definitely survive her. Nothing can happen to him as long as she is alive! She confidently assured us that I could perform the surgery without any worries.

I asked our anaesthetist, Dr Anand, who said that if I was ready to take the risk, he would help me with very light anaesthesia. We requested our friend and cardiologist Dr S.B.Hegde, cardiologist, if he would help us monitor the patient during the surgery. He too was magnanimously co-operative. I called in my brother from Calcutta for the possible bad eventualities. We kept a unit of blood ready. I called in my close friend Dr Venkata Rao, a very successful surgeon colleague of mine, to assist me.

Dr Anand gave a very smooth and effective anaesthesia. I worked as fast as possible but not hurriedly. The prostate adenoma was enucleated and the surgery was over in about 45 minutes. The blood was transfused, and my father was shifted to the ward. We did not have any ICU. I monitored him all through the next 24 hours, and he was quite chirpy by the third day morning.

I was happy to see that my father recovered fast, without any complications. He was very pleased to see the lovely stream of urine he had not seen for years! He came 'home' (above the nursing home) in about eight to ten days and lived a normal life.

My mother passed away around two weeks after this surgery! My father lived for about three years more, and died of a severe third MI.

Some Disappointments

Even as I chronicle my successes, I cannot forget some inevitable sad incidents too. I remember them as vividly as I do my high points. They do make me sad, and I try to pacify myself thinking that, after all, I too am a human being.

'Primum non nocere' is an oft-repeated Latin maxim, which in simple terms means, 'first, do no harm'. Unfortunately, a surgeon's operation begins with a harm (incision) before he heals! On rare occasions, instead of healing, this may even end up with an unintended outcome, sometimes insignificant, sometimes serious, and sometimes even fatal!

Some failures can perhaps be attributed to the lack of facilities like lab, blood bank, equipment, and so on. In the early days of our practice, a lady delivered her baby normally. We were waiting for the placenta to come out. When the placenta did come out, she suddenly bled profusely. There was no blood bank in town, and we could not save her.

Some others were due to advanced pathology, poor health of the patient, associated diseases like uncontrolled diabetes, and so on, like the lady with tuberculous intestinal obstruction described earlier.

Some died despite the best surgery, good facilities and medicines. Some others were so poor financially that they did not have enough resources to cover the expenses of full treatment.

However, there were also some failures due to deficiencies in my techniques or mistakes, though unintended. These happen in every surgeon's life – and end up as their worst, and saddest memories.

One such error was when I performed an operation on a lady, to explore the common bile duct to remove gall stones. After the common duct was clear, I tried to dilate the sphincter in the duodenum so that smaller stones, if any, would pass through. I felt the dilator enter the duodenum, but did not realise that the pancreatic duct might have been injured too. She developed pancreatic fistula. I took the help of a colleague and tried to repair it but could not. Then I referred her to a higher centre, where she died. The husband was rightfully upset with me.

There is another story, this time about a close friend of mine who wanted to be operated upon by me and I alone. I did not want to, as I sincerely felt that he did not need that surgery. I tried very hard to dissuade him by trying to find him very good alternative solutions, and surgeons. But he did not agree, and I had to perform the simple abdominal operation. However, it was an unlucky day for me – or perhaps my fate, as, for the first and the last time in my career, an abdominal mop was left in the abdomen. If it were diagnosed in time after the surgery, my friend could have been saved. But unfortunately, the mop was missed by the experienced ultra-sonologist on two successive occasions; he probably thought, how could an experienced surgeon make such a silly mistake. However, during the third scan, when he finally boldly suggested the presence of a mop, the infection had got out of control and I lost my friend. This became a medico-legal issue, and also a case in the state consumer forum. It affected my practice severely, and career adversely. I realised how vulnerable we surgeons were; even with unintentional mistakes, we become victims of bad publicity by unfavourable media, and of the unscrupulous legal community.

23. The Future

I am 87 years old, as I write this book in 2022. My stars have finally proved that they control me. All of a sudden, my health took a turn for the worse in 2019 (my age 84), making me incapable of most physical activities. The first was a major heart attack, total blockage of the main stent in my heart. It was because of the interventional cardiologist Dr. T.H.Shivshankar's desperate and persistent attempts and success to dislodge the block that I have survived. As I was recovering from it, Covid-19 struck me. Then, there were problems of poly-cythaemia vera (PCV) due to JAK 2 mutation related to blood clotting, and finally there came the gout! I was literally "grounded". The astrologer's prediction could not have been more accurate. Of course, Usha and I retired much earlier, and our nursing home is also closed. But my mind is alert, and my hands are luckily quite steady. So, I am busy pursuing my second dearest pastime – painting! I have completed quite a few oils and water colour paintings.

When I was born in British India, ours was considered to be one of the 'third world countries' and now am in one of the leading nations of the world. I am glad that I chose India over the UK. My father's vision, as also my dream became a reality. Now I am a part of the India, which, having become independent, has prospered, progressed, and advanced technologically in leaps and bounds to become one of the rich nations of the world. Life expectancy in India at the time of Independence was 32 years, now it is 70; maternal mortality was 2000 and now it is 103 per 1,00,000 live births; infant mortality was 150 and it is now 28.7 per 1000 live births. We had just 20 medical colleges with 1500 students then; now we have over 612 colleges and over 91,927 MBBS seats. The number of registered medical practitioners has increased to over 13 lakhs (of that, 10.41 lakh MBBS); hospitals have increased from a mere 7,000 to over 69,000 in public plus private sectors. When I returned from the UK in 1967, our economic situation was such that we were asked to skip a meal once a week; we had to import food grains; now we are the second largest wheat producer of the world. We export milk; we export medicines; we gave free covid vaccines to over 100 neighbouring nations. We have robotic surgery in India, and our laparoscopic surgeons are some of the very best in the world. All this, in a matter of 70 years. My place, Shimoga, which was almost a backward town 50 years ago, now has two medical colleges and multiple corporate hospitals. Shimoga city is now become a tertiary health care centre. I am very proud of all this. In addition, I am happy too, that I could be near our parents in their old age, and see our children settle in life.

We believe that the progress we have made in rural surgery during this period is significant too; more so in our Karnataka state. Laparoscopes, C-arms, labs have gone to rural areas. This progress is solely due to the efforts of, and innovations by rural surgeons on their own! They had to get out of the Western template of a surgeon and create their own identity. Rural surgeons' practices may be off the track, may not be found in textbooks, but they are very effective and useful. I believe that the textbooks contain information about surgery for people in Western countries. It is difficult to find information on surgical techniques suitable for poor Indian conditions. That is why rural surgeons come up with their own innovations, especially suited for Indian patients. Their resilience is tremendous; even when books do not have answers, they somehow manage to deliver good results. I am reminded about an incident that shows how the Indian brain finds simple solutions to problem that others consider complicated. When an earthquake in Sikkim destroyed its road connectivity some years ago, the international agencies needed six weeks to study and then repair the connectivity. It is said that our own Border Roads Organisation repaired it in 19 hours! That is how rural surgery has survived, developed and succeeded over the years, in caring for the rural population irrespective of the total indifference of the academia, medical colleges and other establishments.

I have faith that rural surgery will be improved even further, by the dedication and diligence of current and future rural surgeons. They have the potential to make wondrous changes in the healthcare system. They are the unrecognised, silent healthcare workers in our communities and nation. I salute them.

I have always felt that India will need many more rural surgeons in the future. The Ministry of Health and Family Welfare has reported a 68 percent shortage of specialists (like surgeons, physicians, obstetricians and gynaecologists, paediatricians etc.) in the community health centres nationwide. Lancet Global Health has shown that despite all the progress and increase in the number of healthcare providers, in many parts of India, 32.9 percent of all deaths are from conditions needing surgical care. So, we need more surgeons, that too in small towns and rural areas. Surgery is now considered to be an "indivisible, indispensable part of health care." India has about one surgeon per population of 40,000 (31,560 general surgeons as of 19th May 2017), whereas we need 1 per 5000, and that too easily available! (Lancet Global Health). Surgeons must be accessible within two hours of the emergency to be able to save a life or limb! So, we need more surgeons in rural areas. Attention is needed in improving the district and taluka hospitals; they are the first ports of call for most of the patients. Simple surgical care must be available in every Primary Health Care Centre.

I referred earlier to the potential of rural surgeons. If we put on an Indian cap or turban and think about Indian patients seriously, we can innovatively develop new technologies suited to Indian conditions. The 'Jaipur foot' is one such famous Indian creation. It was conceived especially for Indian farmers who have to 'walk' in the muddy slush of rice fields and even climb trees! Former President of India, the late Sri Abdul Kalam told us at one of our conferences that interaction between orthopaedic surgeons of Nizam Institute of Medical Sciences and the Defence Research and Development Laboratory resulted in the development of Floor Reaction Orthosis (FRO) that reduced the weight of children's callipers from 4 kg to 400 gm! Now the children who were crying and struggling with the heavy lower limb prosthesis could run around happily. Late President Kalam also told us about the cheap cardiac stents developed by the DRDO lab, which cost a fraction of the cost of imported stents and also about the rapid field test kit for detecting typhoid fever in 10 hours as against 10 days taken by the conventional test! Another, more recent famous Indian innovation, is the use of a mosquito net, costing only a couple of rupees, instead of expensive commercial mesh, for the repair of groin hernia. It has revolutionised hernia surgery in developing countries.

The greed of the surgical fraternity helps corporate hospitals to thrive, to such an extent that the small hospitals and nursing homes, which are affordable and patient-friendly, are finding it difficult to survive. Unfortunately, the victims of all this are the common, poor or middle-class patients, and small-town patients.

As said before, despite the great advances India has made, and despite the increase in the number of medical colleges, there is still a need of rural surgeons in towns and rural places. Conscientious surgeons still have opportunities to start their practice in smaller towns; there is demand for small hospitals with modern facilities, but not the type I started with nor like those with corporate philosophy. People have become more prosperous, more knowledgeable, they have Google at their fingertips and have become more 'rights and compensation conscious'. They see newer technologies being used around them and would expect those technologies in their own healthcare too.

A medium-sized hospital with qualified personnel and well equipped with a laboratory, X-ray/ CT scan, primary specialists like a surgeon and an anaesthetist, and a small team comprising a qualified obstetrician, paediatrician and a physician each, may be a working model for a small town. The difficulty would be in finding like-minded persons, and the huge initial investment needed for such ventures. I believe that an individual new surgeon would find it very difficult to find resources for this, and to survive despite the predatory corporate hospitals.

The government needs to wake up to the reality that Bharat needs its own technology for rural health care as shown by present practicing surgeons. It needs to encourage those that venture to take up rural surgery with assistance and finances.

However, I believe that a general practitioner (family physician who makes house calls) and a general surgeon (who will be the first surgical specialist to call upon, and to decide future management of the condition) will always be the most important pillars of healthcare at all the times.

We are notorious for enacting laws before making the country ready for it. We enforced pollution control laws long before we knew the correct methods of waste disposal. We introduced blood bank rules in 1992-93, even before we had enough blood banks. Even now, twenty years later, UDBT, that is, the old method of collecting blood from the donor and transfusing it into the patient, needs to be used in many parts of the country. It has saved thousands of lives. I believe that UDBT is the only way of saving lives in those areas. The new concept of 'walking blood banks' is very good too. They both must be permitted by law.

We need to produce more surgeons, anaesthetists, nurses, and such healthcare professionals, to meet the rising demand in rural areas. We need special training centres for those surgeons who choose to go the small towns and rural areas. Even more important is teaching communication skills to win over the confidence of the patients and relatives. I believe that lack of this skill is one of the reasons of physical assaults on doctors. Most of the developed countries have training centres for rural physicians as described earlier. And yet despite the wonderful progress that India has made in many fields, a rural surgeon may still have to overcome some unexpected shortcomings like I had to. But for those surgeons who love surgery, countryside, fresh air, and a quiet simple life, there is nothing like a small-town practice.

24. Sharing Our Success

This book is about our surgical practice in Shimoga. It is much more than the story of our practice only. There have been some very important people who were a part of the team and without whom our practice would not have been as successful as it has been. I wish to share our success with them.

The following four were the important faces in our hospital…

Govinda Gudimane joined us as a compounder (unqualified). But he learnt all that was there to learn in OT work, nursing, assisting at surgeries, keeping inventories of goods, and much more. He was the Jack-of-all-trades for most of the hospital work. His devotion to his job was fantastic.

Nurse Savitri had no formal nursing training. But her clinical acumen has saved us on many an occasion. She would remember the medical-clinical, social and even financial histories of almost all our patients!

Nurse Jayamary was also 'unqualified' though trained by us. She had a lot of empathy for patients. Nurse Raheema, though a graduate, was also an 'unqualified' nurse. She became an expert in OT techniques and at assistance at surgeries with training!

All four excelled in their work, many a times stepping beyond the line of duty, so much so that their names represented the hospital! They managed all aspects of nursing and administration, in their own ways. They were the soul of the Dutta Hospital so to say. Many patients came asking for them and not us.

Dr Anand worked as an anaesthetist with us for many years. His bold ways and management of all types of patients was admirable. His methods did not fit into any standard protocols – he created protocols to suit each patient. In my opinion, he was a perfect rural anaesthetist. He boldly anaesthetised my 89-year-old father despite his high cardiac risks, when all other leading anaesthetists had refused to come near him. He has contributed immensely to our success.

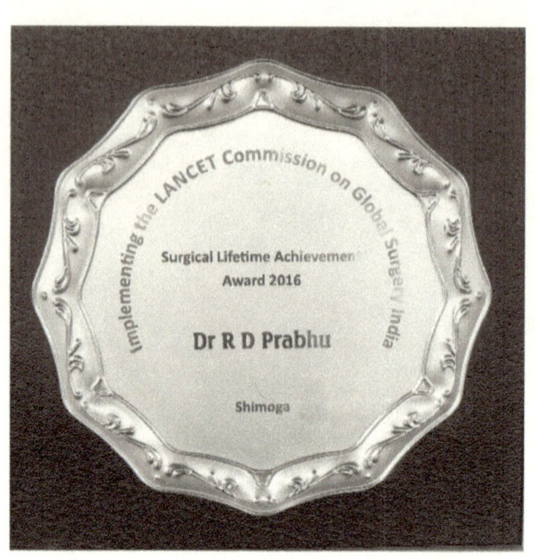

Surgical Lifetime Achievement Award 2016 by Lancet Global Health

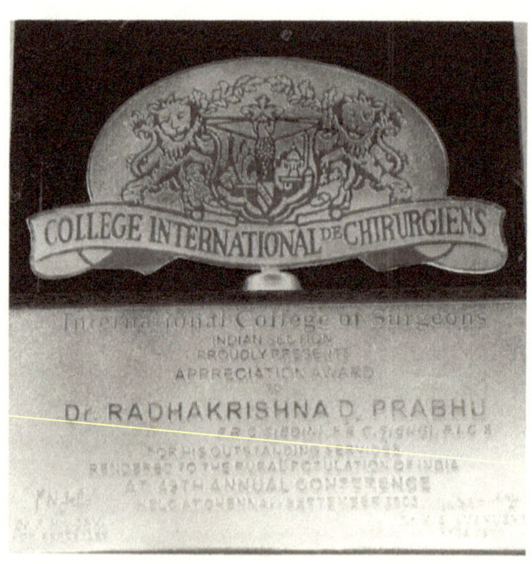

Appreciation Award by the International College of Surgeons, Indian Section 2003
For Outstanding Service rendered to Rural Population of India

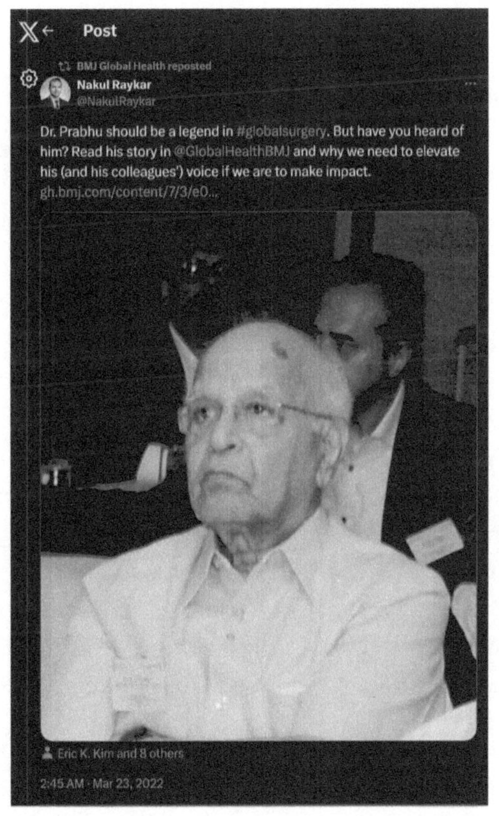

Dr. R. D. Prabhu.
FRCS(Eng), FRCS(Edin), FICS(IS), FARSI

Past president, ARSI,
Past President, IFRS,
Past chairman, KSC,ASI,
Past R.I.Officer, Rotary International

BMJ Article

Rural surgery as global surgery before global surgery

Eric K Kim[1][2], Rohini Dutta[3][4], Nobhojit Roy[4],Nakul Raykar[2][5][6]

Rural surgeons should be at the helm of global surgery efforts, yet we rarely hear from these pioneers. While high-income country (HIC) surgeons leverage their institutional power to publish in high-impact journals and advance their careers, rural surgeons tirelessly tackle the daily struggles of delivering quality surgical care in low-resource settings. Because of the current power structures within global surgery, the toil of rural surgeons is left out and remains unrecognised. With conscientious efforts to make global surgery more inclusive, however, we can harness the collective knowledge of rural surgeons who frequently devise creative, actionable solutions that can more immediately address barriers to care in low resource settings.

Long before the term global surgery was conceived, rural surgeons were striving to secure healthcare for the 5 billion individuals who lack access to safe, affordable, surgical and anaesthesia care. Beyond their role as clinicians, rural surgeons also have a long track record of advocating for their patients, who are usually the most socioeconomically disadvantaged of their region. This focus on equity and advocacy is recognised as a core feature of global health and global surgery. One example of a rural surgeon who exemplifies these values is Dr Radhakrishna D Prabhu. Born in Ankola, India and trained in Mumbai and the UK, Dr Prabhu returned to Shimoga, India with a mission to serve the country's marginalised rural population. Despite the stark economic disparities between Shimoga and the UK, he remained undaunted. Recognising that his patients would simply never get the operations they needed unless he was well-versed in a variety of surgical subspecialties, Dr Prabhu practiced broadly. In his career, he has performed 36 of the 44 WHO Essential Surgeries (figure 1), in addition to many more not on the list. Dr Prabhu is not alone in his clinical expanse. In a survey he conducted in 1986, he demonstrated that 66% of rural surgeons performed surgeries in more than three surgical subspecialties. To overcome material and infrastructural constraints, he relied on his ingenuity. Facing severe blood shortages, Dr Prabhu pioneered a technology that we now know as autologous transfusion, the practice of collecting and re-transfusing one's own blood. Another example of such resourcefulness is Dr Ravi Tongaonkar, an Indian rural surgeon and friend of Dr Prabhu, who invented the idea of using sterilised mosquito nets as a cost-effective alternative to commercial hernia mesh. This innovation from rural surgery demonstrated non-inferiority to commercial meshes in the rates of hernia recurrence and complications in a randomised controlled trial published in the New England Journal of Medicine. 8 As the predecessor and embodiment of global surgery, rural surgery has numerous lessons to impart. To learn from the wisdom of rural surgery, we propose the following steps for the academic global surgery community:

First, global surgery conferences and societies must actively recruit and provide platforms for representatives of low middle-income country (LMIC) rural surgery. Similar to how the National Institute of Health vowed to end all-male panels, or 'manels', 9 global health organisations need to avoid all-HIC panels and executive boards and include more representatives from LMICs in leadership. The well-documented under-representation of LMIC attendees at global health conferences represents a missed opportunity. 10 LMIC speakers and panellists will highlight the issues they face as well as successful solutions, allowing HIC and

LMIC surgeons to learn, exchange knowledge and forge new partnerships. Additionally, hosting conferences in 'visa-friendly' countries or LMICs themselves can ease a major barrier to attendance. 10 HIC organisations must increase the amount of scholarships and grants to support rural surgeons to engage in global surgery events, as the costs of registration fees, travel and lodging are prohibitively high.

Second, while advocacy in global surgery has been dominated by the important work of incorporating surgical care into the health systems frameworks of national and international governing bodies, we argue that a broader frame is necessary for global surgery advocacy. For example, rural surgeons practice a wide scope of surgeries spanning multiple surgical specialties, as detailed below:

List Of Essential Skills For Rural Surgery
　Dental
　　Dental Extraction
　　Drainage of dental abscess
　　Treatment for caries
　Obstetric, gynecological and family planning
　　Normal delivery
　　Caesarean birth
　　Vacuum extraction or forceps delivery
　　Ectopic pregnancy
　　Manual vacuum aspiration and dilation and curettage
　　Tubal ligation
　　Vasectomy
　　Hysterectomy for uterine rupture or intractable post-partum haemorrhage
　　Visual inspection with acetic acid and cryotherapy for precancerous cervical lesions
　　Repair obstetric fistula
　General surgical
　　Drainage of superficial abscess
　　Male circumcision
　　Repair of perforations (perforated peptic ulcer, typhoid ileal perforation, etc)
　　Appendectomy

Bowel obstruction
Colostomy
Gallbladder disease (including emergency surgery for acute cholecystitis)
Hernia (including incarceration)
Hydrocelectomy
Relief of urinary obstruction: catheterisation or suprapubic cystostomy (tube into bladder through skin)

Injury
Resuscitation with basic life support measures
Suturing laceration
Management of non-displaced fractures
Resuscitation with advanced life support measures, including surgical airway†
Tube thoracostomy (chest drain)
Trauma laparotomy
Fracture reduction Irrigation and debridement of open fractures
Placement of external fixator: use of traction
Escharotomy or fasciotomy (cutting of constricting tissue to relieve pressure from swelling)
Trauma-related amputations
Skin grafting
Burr hole

Congenital
Cleft lip and palate repair
Club foot repair
Shunt for hydrocephalus
Repair of anorectal malformations and Hirschsprung's disease

Visual impairment
Cataract extraction and insertion of intraocular lens
Eyelid surgery for trachoma

Non-trauma orthopaedic
Drainage of septic arthritis
Debridement of osteomyelitis

Note : Underlined are EMERGENCY PROCEDURES

Without formal recognition of the broad scope of practice necessitated in these contexts, rural global surgeons like Dr Prabhu feel they perform these life-saving surgeries at great personal legal risk. Professional governing bodies and academic surgical societies can establish pathways for this recognition, which may include certification in different procedures and specialties, and global surgery advocates should actively lobby for more explicit protection from governments of surgeons in low-resource communities with a broad scope of practice.

Finally, before a global surgery trainee learns about Dr Prabhu or Dr Tongaonkar, hey will more likely learn the names of HIC academic surgeons championing the cause of global surgery. Because the visibility of LMIC global surgeons is abysmally low, the trainee may envision these HIC professors as their global surgery role models. By publicising the works of physicians like Dr Prabhu, the academic global surgery community can help change this narrative. It can promote the research, advocacy and viewpoints of global surgeons in LMICs and relate different avenues through which the broader community can learn.

We hope that, in turn, trainees will realise that rural surgeons like Dr Prabhu are the true masters in global surgery and are inspired to take up the mantle and bring quality surgical care to the patients who need it the most.

Summary

1. Rural surgeons in low-income and middle-income countries have been providing life-saving surgeries to underserved patients in low-resource settings for many years, long before the term global surgery became popular.
2. Rural surgeons like Dr Radhakrishna D Prabhu, who perform essential surgeries across multiple specialties and use cost-saving innovations to make surgery affordable,

have valuable knowledge that can help and guide global surgery efforts.

3. Rural surgeons should be leading the field of global surgery, but they have long been neglected by the academic global surgery community.

4. The academic global surgery community can elevate the voices of rural surgeons by actively seeking and providing resources for their engagement in academic opportunities and lending support to rural surgeons' research and policy agenda.

(Acknowledgements We sincerely thank Dr Radhakrishna D Prabhu for allowing us to read and draw inspiration from excerpts of his soon-to- be released memoir as a rural surgeon in India and sharing his insights and experiences that shaped this commentary.)

Author affiliations

1 University of California San Francisco School of Medicine, San Francisco, California, USA

2 Program in Global Surgery and Social Change, Harvard Medical School, Boston, Massachusetts, USA

3 Christian Medical College and Hospital, Ludhiana, India

4 World Health Organization Collaborating Centre for Research in Surgical Care Delivery in Low-and-Middle Income Countries, Mumbai, India

5 Center for Surgery and Public Health, Brigham and Women's Hospital, Boston, Massachusetts, USA

6 Trauma, Emergency Surgery, Surgical Critical Care, Brigham and Women's Hospital, Boston, MA, 02215

Published by **BMJ. BMJ Global Health 2022;7:e008222. doi:10.1136/bmjgh-2021-008222 on 22 March 2022**

What Readers Say

Yes, it will be on our distribution and reading list for our young Global Surgery fellows program in India. Well done, Dr. Prabhu!

Dr. Nabhojit Roy. Lancet Global Health

Dr. Prabhu, what a delightful message – congratulations!!!!

I will surely purchase the book through Amazon India and pick it up the next time I am in India. I will bring back a few copies for our PGSSC team as well.

Must feel good to have the book complete! It will be a great resource and inspiration for many to come.

Dr. Nakul Raykar, Harvard University, Lancet Global Health

Dr Prabhu's description of tackling some of the unexpected surgical problems is truly fascinating. They may sound crude and unorthodox to the present day rural surgeons even but they were helpful. I am sure many of the rural surgeons had to tackle such problems. Dr Prabhu's sugar dressing for infected wounds and the explanation for its effectiveness are worthy for trying. I learned Ghee and honey dressing from Dr T Udwadia and found it to be very effective for infective wounds.

Dr. S. K. Baasu, Past president ARSI

I should have written to you earlier since I had finished reading
your book in a single setting. You are a PIONEER in the true
sense of the word. Starting from scratch you built a hospital to suit
the needs of the poor and the middle class group of patients of the
community. The rich will always go towards the cities. But your
group of patients had at least those days a deep sense of gratitude.
This is as you have rightly pointed out disappearing very quickly in
tier 3 cities and smaller towns. A very unfortunate
development indeed. The corporate culture is ruining the
medical practice of this country. Its tentacles are spreading far and
wide.

Dr. C.R.Ballal Prof. K.M.C.Mangalore

Having read & re-read your book, what struck me most was the
simple, unpretentious & down-to-earth narration. When you say
that a lot has been achieved, but some things could've been better,
I could feel your anguish. It is unfortunate that a system can ignore
all the good a person has done while judging a rare, unwitting error.
I can imagine, in a small town like Shimoga, the odds you & your
young doctor wife must have faced in setting up a practice, what
with no trained nurses, no anaesthetist & the erratic power supply -
which you have presented so humorously despite the seriousness
of your situation! It takes a lot of courage, determination &
dedication to the job in hand to keep going & not be deterred by
adversities.

Sarala Mahale

www.ingramcontent.com/pod-product-compliance
Lightning Source LLC
Chambersburg PA
CBHW031623170726

47990CB00016B/346